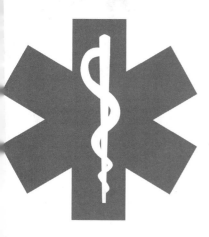

Medical Case Studies for the Paramedic

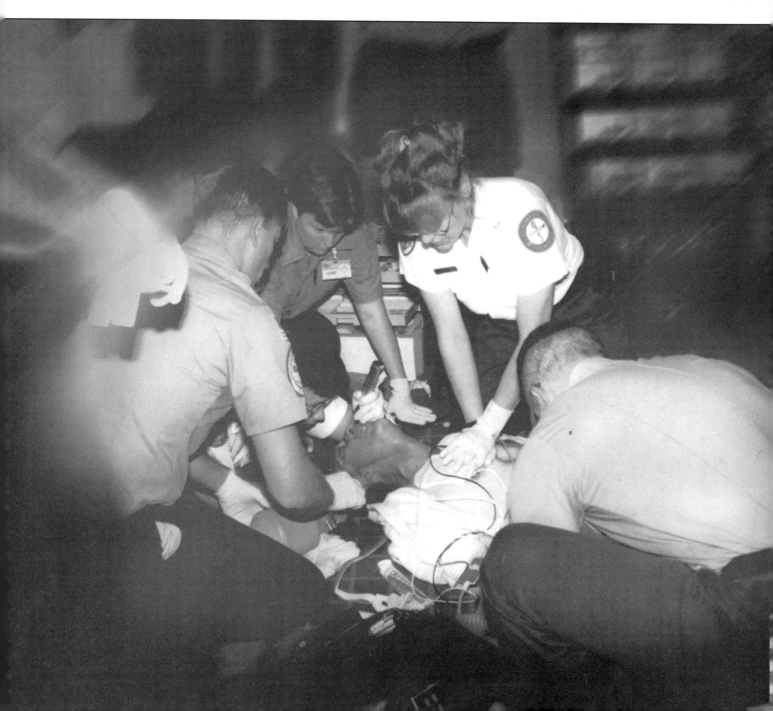

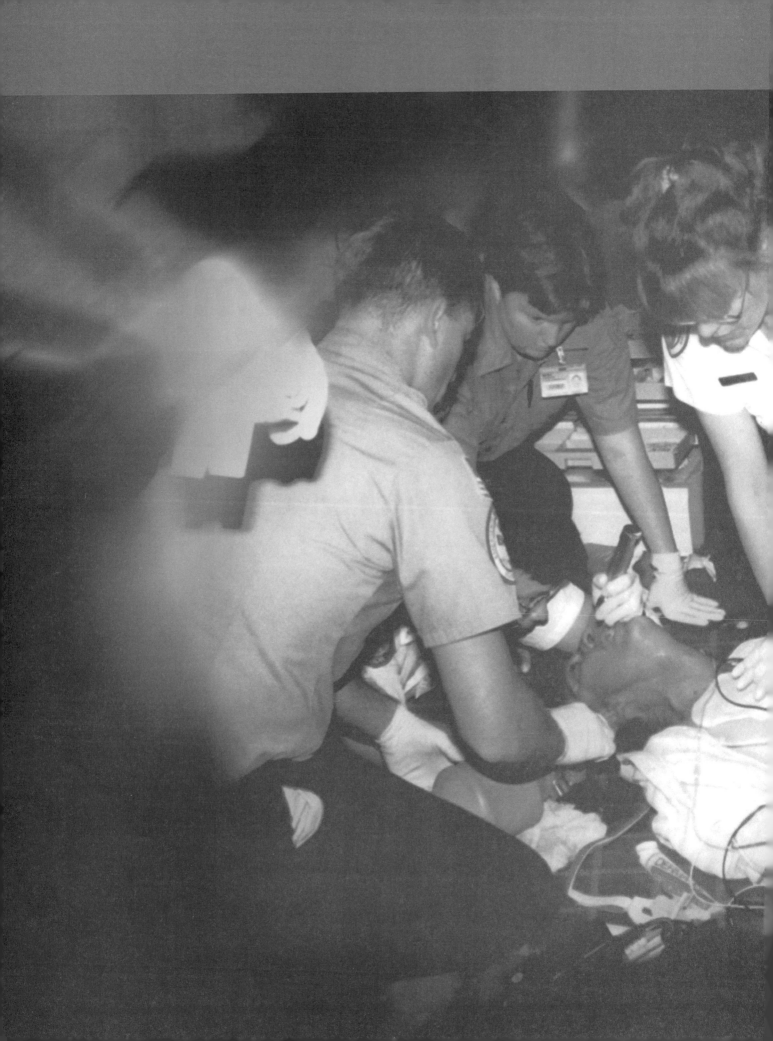

Medical Case Studies for the Paramedic

Stephen J. Rahm, NREMT-P
Author
Kendall County EMS Training Institute
Boerne, Texas

Andrew N. Pollak, MD, EMT-P, FAAOS
Medical Editor
University of Maryland School of Medicine
Baltimore, Maryland

JONES AND BARTLETT PUBLISHERS
Sudbury, Massachusetts
BOSTON   TORONTO   LONDON   SINGAPORE

Jones and Bartlett Publishers

World Headquarters
40 Tall Pine Drive
Sudbury, MA 01776
978-443-5000
info@jbpub.com
www.jbpub.com

Jones and Bartlett Publishers Canada
2406 Nikanna Rd.
Mississauga, ON L5C 2W6
Canada

Jones and Bartlett Publishers International
Barb House, Barb Mews
London W6 7PA
United Kingdom

Production Credits
Chief Executive Officer: Clayton Jones
Chief Operating Officer: Don W. Jones, Jr.
President: Robert W. Holland, Jr.
V.P., Design and Production: Anne Spencer
V.P., Sales and Marketing: William Kane
V.P., Manufacturing and Inventory Control: Therese Bräuer
Publisher, Public Safety Group: Kimberly Brophy
Associate Managing Editor: Carol E. Brewer
Production Assistant: Carolyn F. Rogers
Director of Marketing: Alisha Weisman
Cover and Text Design: Anne Spencer
Cover Photo © Eddie Sperling
Chapter 9 Opener © Craig Jackson/In the Dark Photography
Chapter 20 Opener © Joel Gordon 1990
Composition: Jason Miranda
Printing and Binding: Courier Stoughton

American Academy of Orthopaedic Surgeons

This textbook is intended solely as a guide to the appropriate procedures to be employed when rendering emergency care to the sick and injured. It is not intended as a statement of the standards of care required in any particular situation, because circumstances and the patient's physical condition can vary widely from one emergency to another. Nor is it intended that this textbook shall in any way advise emergency personnel concerning legal authority to perform the activities or procedures discussed. Such local determinations should be made only with the aid of legal counsel.

ISBN: 0-7637-2581-1

Library of Congress Cataloging-in-Publication Data

Rahm, Stephen J.
 Medical case studies for the paramedic / Stephen J. Rahm.— 1st ed.
  p. ; cm.
 ISBN 0-7637-2581-1 (pbk. : alk. paper)
 1. Medical emergencies—Case studies.
 [DNLM: 1. Emergency Treatment—methods—Case Reports. 2. Emergency Treatment—methods—Problems and Exercises. 3. Emergency Medical Technicians—education—Case Reports. 4. Emergency Medical Technicians—education—Problems and Exercises. WB 18.2 R147m 2004] I. Title.
 RC86.9.R346 2004
 616.02'5—dc22

                    2004000146

Printed in the United States of America
08 07 06 05 04   10 9 8 7 6 5 4 3 2 1

CONTENTS

CHAPTER PREVIEW

Text Resources

Medical Case Studies for the Paramedic contains 20 case studies representing a variety of medical emergencies. Each case study follows a logical and systematic approach to patient assessment and management. Paramedic students apply knowledge from initial training to real-life scenarios as they complete the case studies and answer corresponding questions.

CASE STUDY

2

68-Year-Old Male with Difficulty Breathing

At 6:45 am, you receive a call to an assisted-living center at 1402 Donaldson Ave for a 68-year-old male with breathing difficulty. Your response time to the scene is approximately 5 to 7 minutes. First responders arrive shortly before you and your partner.

You arrive at the scene at 6:51 am. As you enter the patient's room, you find him sitting in a chair with a blanket up to his waist. He is in obvious respiratory distress and is noticeably pale and diaphoretic. You perform an initial assessment (**Table 2-1**) as an attendant in the assisted-living center retrieves the patient's medical records.

Table 2-1 Initial Assessment

Level of Consciousness	Responds minimally when spoken to
Chief Complaint	Difficulty breathing, altered mental status
Airway and Breathing	Respirations are rapid and profoundly labored; blood-tinged secretions are flowing from his mouth
Circulation	Radial pulses are absent; carotid pulse is rapid, weak, and irregular; skin is cool, pale, and diaphoretic

---

1. What initial management is indicated for this patient?

After moving the patient to the floor, your partner and a first responder ing the patient's airway. Meanwhile, you perform a focused history and examination (**Table 2-2**). The attendant, who has returned with the pati records, provides you with the information you need.

Table 2-2 Focused History and Physical Examination

Onset	"We first noticed his condition about 6 hours ago, suddenly worsened."
Associated Symptoms	"He complained of chest pain yesterday, but refused to allow us to call an ambulance."
Evidence of Trauma	None
Interventions Prior to EMS Arrival	"We moved him from his bed to the chair, where we thought he would be more comfortable."
Seizures	"I haven't seen any seizures."
Fever	"No, he has not been running a fever."
Chest Exam	Intercostal retractions, sporadic chest wall movement
Breath Sounds	Coarse rhonchi are audible in all lung fields without a stethoscope.
Blood Glucose	140 mg/dL
Pupils	Dilated and slow to react

A cardiac monitor is attached and a 6-second rhythm strip is obtained (**Figure 2-1**). You assess the cardiac rhythm as your partner and the first responder continue to manage the patient's airway.

■ **Figure 2-1** Your patient's cardiac rhythm.

---

2. What is your interpretation of this cardiac rhythm?

Your partner advises you that the patient is now continuously producing blood-tinged secretions and his respirations are deteriorating. A first responder inserts a nasopharyngeal airway and preoxygenates the patient with a bag-valve-mask (BVM) device as your partner prepares to perform endotracheal (ET) intubation. You obtain baseline vital signs and a SAMPLE history (**Table 2-3**). You retrieve the patient's medical history information from his medical records.

Table 2-3 Baseline Vital Signs and SAMPLE History

Blood Pressure	78/48 mm Hg
Pulse	100 beats/min, irregular and thready
Respirations	Ventilated with a BVM device at a rate of 15 breaths/min
Oxygen Saturation	94% (ventilated with 100% oxygen)
Signs and Symptoms	Altered mental status, hypotension, and pulmonary edema
Allergies	Meperidine hydrochloride (Demerol) and promethazine hydrochloride (Phenergan)
Medications	Digoxin (Lanoxin), furosemide (Lasix), potassium chloride (K-Dur), enalapril maleate (Vasotec), and warfarin sodium (Coumadin)
Pertinent Past History	Congestive heart failure, hypertension
Last Oral Intake	The patient has refused to eat for the past 2 days.
Events Leading to Present Illness	Complained of chest pain yesterday

3. What is your field impression of this patient?

Each case begins with a thorough case presentation.
Initial Assessment information is presented in a table.

Baseline Vital Signs and SAMPLE History information is presented in a table.

Fill-in-the-blank questions are interspersed throughout the case for students to answer as they read.

Focused History and Physical Examination information is presented in a table.

High-quality rhythm strips show the patient's cardiac rhythm.

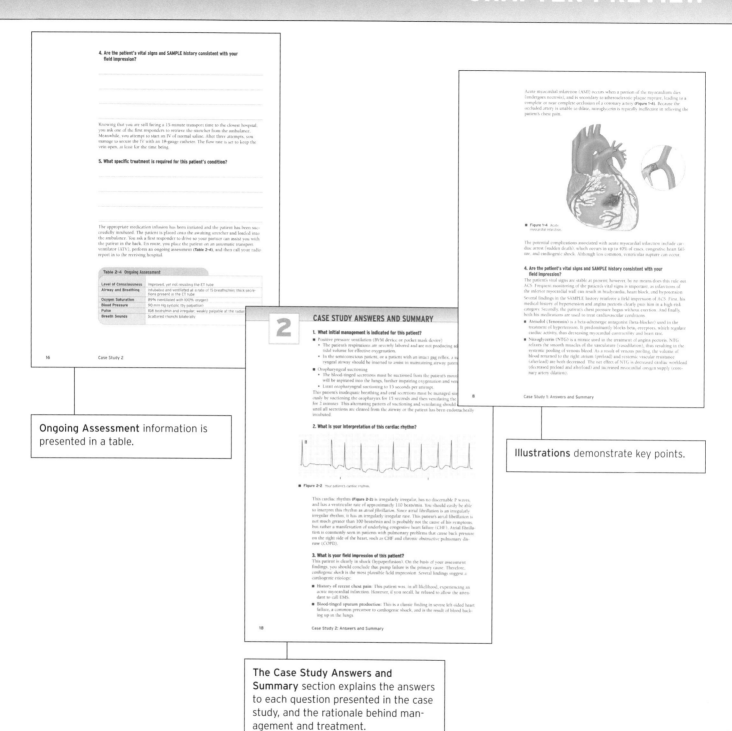

Ongoing Assessment information is presented in a table.

Illustrations demonstrate key points.

The Case Study Answers and Summary section explains the answers to each question presented in the case study, and the rationale behind management and treatment.

Other titles in the Case Studies series include:

Trauma Case Studies for the Paramedic

ISBN: 0-7637-2583-8

Pediatric Case Studies for the Paramedic

ISBN: 0-7637-2582-X

Jones & Bartlett Publishers would like to thank the following people for reviewing this text.

Jeffrey K. Benes, BS, EMT-P
Central DuPage Hospital
Winfield, Illinois

Julie Chase
Angel Fire Fire Department
Angel Fire, New Mexico

Daniel Donahue
Paradise Valley Community College
Phoenix, Arizona

Randy Hardick, BA, NREMT-P
Avera McKennan School of Emergency Medical Services
Sioux Falls, South Dakota

Sandra Dunn Hartley, MS, CP
Pensacola Junior College
Pensacola, Florida

Mark A. Huckaby, NREMTP
Grant Medical Center LifeLink
Columbus, Ohio

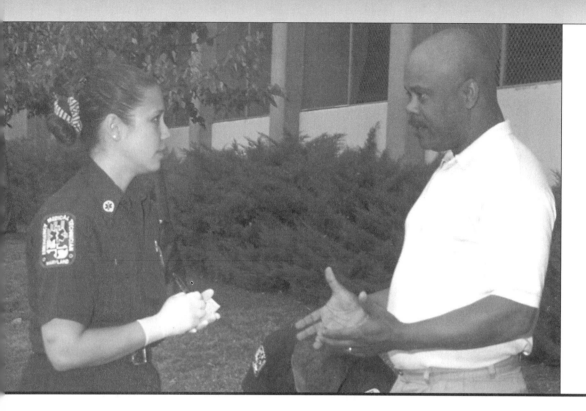

Introduction

Medical Case Studies for the Paramedic contains 20 case studies representing a variety of medical emergencies, some more common than others, that the paramedic may encounter in the field. The objectives for each of the case studies in this book are as follows:

- Describe the appropriate initial management based on initial assessment findings.
- Interpret the patient's cardiac rhythm and determine whether a correlation exists between the rhythm and the patient's condition.
- Formulate a field impression based on the patient's signs and symptoms and findings of the focused history and physical examination.
- Determine whether the patient's vital sign values and SAMPLE history are consistent with your established field impression.
- Identify specific treatment required for the patient's condition.
- Determine whether further treatment is required following reassessment of the patient.
- On the basis of the patient's condition, identify any special considerations for care.

How to Use This Book

Medical Case Studies for the Paramedic is intended to reinforce the importance of a systematic patient assessment and management approach to paramedic students by presenting them with medical emergencies they are likely to encounter in the field. This book should be used as an additional resource for the paramedic student to test newly gained knowledge and prepare for examinations; it should not be used in place of a primary paramedic textbook.

Each case study will begin by presenting you with dispatch information, just as you would receive on an actual call, and a general impression of the patient upon arriving at the scene. Then, as the case progresses, pertinent patient information will be provided, interspersed with a series of standardized questions designed to assess your ability in correlating specific signs and symptoms with a particular medical condition and providing the appropriate treatment.

A suggested method for using this book is to read each part of the case, and then, in the area provided, answer the question that follows in as much detail as possible prior to reading the next part of the case. Your detailed response to the questions will help reinforce your knowledge of the material. Continue this until you have read all of the information and answered all of the case study questions. You may then compare your answers to those outlined in the case summary that immediately follows each case.

The case summary provides answers to the questions asked within the case, as well as additional enrichment information, to include the following:

- Additional signs and symptoms commonly associated with the patient's condition.
- The relevance, if any, of the patient's cardiac rhythm to the condition.
- Information and justification for each treatment modality.
- Specific information regarding the patient's prescribed medications.
- Basic pathophysiology of the patient's condition.

Treatment Guidelines

The treatment recommendations contained within this book conform to the current standards of care as outlined in the following:

- US DOT EMT-Paramedic National Standard Curriculum, revised 1998
- American Heart Association Guidelines and Algorithms, revised 2000
- Brain Trauma Foundation (BTF), 2003

Additional treatment or variations in treatment may be required for each of the conditions presented in this book. As with the management of any patient, the paramedic must conform to the protocols inherent to their EMS system, and should contact medical control as needed.

Body Substance Isolation (BSI) Precautions

Strict adherence to proper body substance isolation (BSI) precautions is of paramount importance when managing any patient. Throughout each of the case studies presented in this book, it is assumed that the proper BSI precautions are being followed at all times.

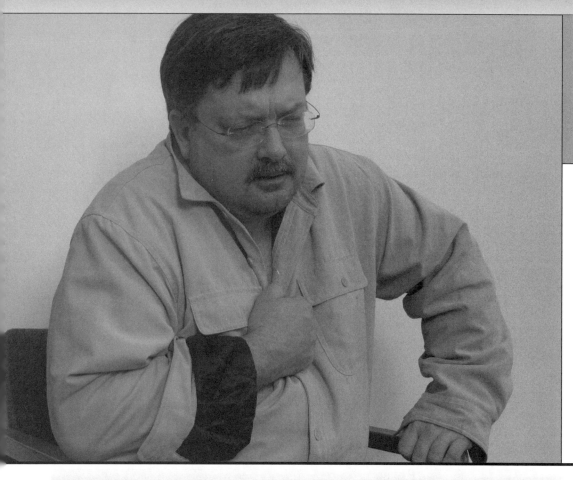

1

49-Year-Old Male with Chest Pressure

At 2:35 pm, you are dispatched to an office building at 124 South Elm Ave for a 49-year-old male patient with chest pressure. Your response time to the scene is 7 minutes.

Upon arriving at the scene, you are greeted at the front door of the office building by a female coworker. As she is escorting you to the patient, she tells you that he took his heart medicine, but is still in a lot of pain. You find the patient sitting in a chair in the front lobby of the office building. He has a fearful look, is clenching his fist against his chest, and is noticeably diaphoretic. After introducing yourself, you perform an initial assessment **(Table 1-1)**.

Table 1-1 Initial Assessment

Level of Consciousness	Patient is conscious and alert to person, place, and time.
Chief Complaint	"I'm having a lot of pressure in my chest, and I'm sick to my stomach."
Airway and Breathing	Airway is patent; respirations are normal.
Circulation	Radial pulse is normal–strong and regular; skin is pale, cool, and diaphoretic.

1. What initial management is indicated for this patient?

_____

_____

_____

_____

The appropriate initial management has been provided to the patient. A cardiac monitor is applied, which reveals a normal sinus rhythm at 70 beats/min in lead II.

Your partner quickly retrieves the stretcher from the ambulance as you perform a focused history and physical examination **(Table 1-2)**.

Table 1-2 Focused History and Physical Examination

Onset	"This pain began suddenly."
Provocation/Palliation	"No matter what I do, this pain will not stop!"
Quality	"It's pressure, not really pain."
Radiation/Referred Pain	"The pain stays in my chest."
Severity	"7" on a scale of 0 to 10
Time	"This started about an hour ago."
Interventions Prior to EMS Arrival	"I've had 3 sprays of my nitroglycerin."
Chest Exam	No obvious trauma, chest wall moves symmetrically
Breath Sounds	Clear and equal bilaterally
Jugular Veins	Normal

The patient is placed supine on the stretcher, and a 12-lead ECG is obtained. After you examine the ECG **(Figure 1-1)**, you and your partner agree that the patient requires immediate transport to the hospital.

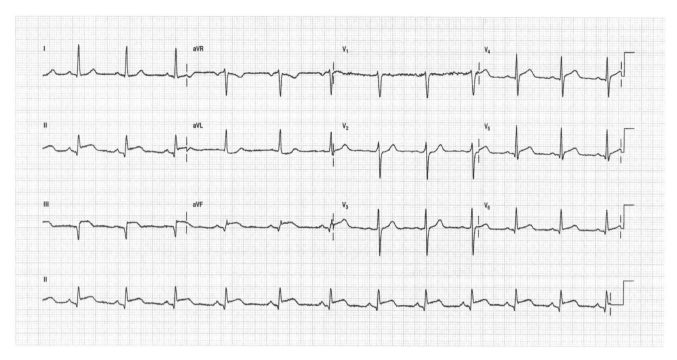

■ **Figure 1-1** Your patient's 12-lead ECG.

2. What is your interpretation of this cardiac rhythm?

_____

_____

_____

_____

Your partner initiates an IV of normal saline and sets the flow rate to keep the vein open (KVO). Meanwhile, you obtain the patient's baseline vital signs and a SAMPLE history **(Table 1-3)**.

Table 1-3 Baseline Vital Signs and SAMPLE History	
Blood Pressure	134/84 mm Hg
Pulse	74 beats/min, strong and regular
Respirations	18 breaths/min and unlabored
Oxygen Saturation	98% (on 100% oxygen)
Signs and Symptoms	Chest pressure, diaphoresis, and nausea
Allergies	"I am allergic to codeine and penicillin."
Medications	Atenolol (Tenormin), nitroglycerin
Pertinent Past History	Hypertension and angina pectoris
Last Oral Intake	"I had a sandwich and coffee 2 hours ago."
Events Leading to Present Illness	"I was sitting at my desk working on a manuscript when the pain began."

3. What is your field impression of this patient?

_____

_____

_____

_____

4. Are the patient's vital signs and SAMPLE history consistent with your field impression?

_____

_____

_____

_____

The patient tells you that his chest pressure has not improved, even after taking 3 nitroglycerin treatments. He also tells you that he has a "pounding headache," which usually happens after he takes his nitroglycerin.

5. What specific treatment is required for this patient's condition?

_____

_____

_____

_____

You initiate specific treatment for the patient's condition. Within 5 minutes after this treatment, he describes his chest pressure as a "3" (previously a 7). After obtaining the patient's blood pressure again (118/70 mm Hg), you load the patient into the ambulance, begin transport to the hospital, and conduct an ongoing assessment en route **(Table 1-4)**.

Table 1-4 Ongoing Assessment

Level of Consciousness	Conscious and alert to person, place, and time
Airway and Breathing	Respirations, 18 breaths/min and unlabored
Oxygen Saturation	98% (on 100% oxygen)
Blood Pressure	116/74 mm Hg
Pulse	86 beats/min, strong and regular
Chest Pain	"3" on a scale of 0 to 10
ECG	Normal sinus rhythm (in lead II)

6. Is further treatment required for this patient?

_____

_____

_____

_____

Further assessment and treatment is provided as needed throughout transport. You call in your radio report to the receiving hospital and give your estimated time of arrival of approximately 6 minutes.

7. Are there any special considerations for this patient?

_____

_____

_____

Upon arrival at the emergency department, you give your verbal report to the attending physician and present him with the 12-lead ECG obtained in the field. The physician orders another 12-lead ECG, which confirms the presence of acute myocardial infarction.

Following further assessment in the emergency department, the patient is administered an IV bolus of reteplase (Retavase) as well as infusions of heparin and nitroglycerin. Within 30 minutes he is pain-free and is admitted to the coronary intensive care unit. One week later, the patient is transferred to a cardiac care rehabilitation facility, where he fully recovered.

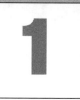

CASE STUDY ANSWERS AND SUMMARY

1. What initial management is indicated for this patient?

- **100% supplemental oxygen via nonrebreathing mask**
  - The patient's respirations are adequate (normal rate and quality); therefore, positive pressure ventilatory support is not required at this time.
  - Oxygen is the first drug administered to any patient with chest pain/pressure, and should be given as soon as possible.

- **Aspirin 160 to 325 mg PO**
  - Aspirin (ASA), or acetylsalicylic acid, should be given as soon as possible to patients with chest pain or pressure suggestive of a cardiac etiology.
  - Aspirin blocks the production of thromboxane A_2, thus inhibiting platelet aggregation. This effect limits propogation of any microemboli that may exist due to plaque rupture within the coronary arteries.
  - To achieve the fastest therapeutic blood level, the patient should be instructed to chew the aspirin prior to swallowing it.
  - If the patient has any known bleeding diathesis (eg, hemophilia), or has a known hypersensitivity to salicylates, aspirin should not be administered.

2. What is your interpretation of this cardiac rhythm?

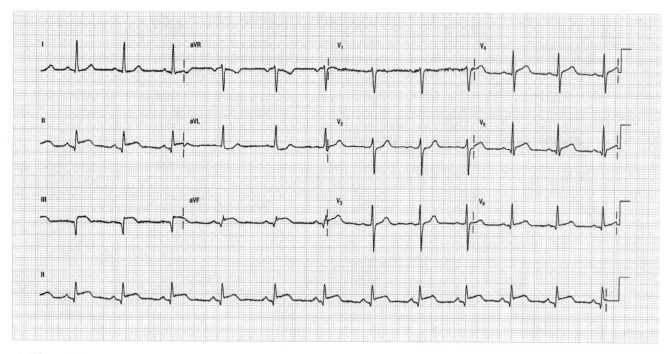

■ **Figure 1-2** Your patient's 12-lead ECG.

The underlying rhythm is a sinus rhythm, with a ventricular rate of approximately 60 to 70 beats/min **(Figure 1-2)**. ST-segment elevation is shown in leads II, III, and aVF (inferior leads), as well as in leads V_4 to V_6 (lateral leads). There is reciprocal ST-segment depression in lead aVL (lateral lead). The changes in this ECG are consistent with *inferolateral wall myocardial infarction!*

Q waves are beginning to form in the inferior leads, which could suggest an old inferior wall infarction, or, more likely, an infarction that is only a few hours old. Q waves without ST-segment changes would be more indicative of an old myocardial infarction.

3. What is your field impression of this patient?

This patient is experiencing an *acute coronary syndrome (ACS)*, a term used to describe either unstable angina or acute myocardial infarction. In the case of this patient, we have already established an acute myocardial infarction by the grossly abnormal 12-lead ECG. The following pertinent findings would suggest an acute coronary syndrome, even in the absence of a 12-lead ECG:

- **Prescribed nitroglycerin** is given to patients with coronary artery disease, so we know this patient has a history of cardiac disease.

- **Chest pain or pressure**, present in about 80% of all cases of acute coronary syndrome, is commonly described by the patient by holding a clenched fist tightly against the chest (Levine's sign).

- **Unrelieved chest pain or pressure** despite the administration of nitroglycerin or other palliating factors (eg, rest) is consistent with unstable angina or myocardial infarction.

- **Diaphoresis** indicates a sympathetic nervous system discharge and subsequent activation of the sweat glands. In some patients, sudden diaphoresis may be the only presenting sign of ACS.

- **Feeling of impending doom.** Frighteningly enough, people know when something bad is happening to them. The fearful look that this patient has should be taken seriously.

Angina pectoris occurs when the myocardium is transiently deprived of oxygen (ischemia). Although coronary vasospasm can cause angina (Prinzmetal's angina), it is most often the result of atherosclerotic coronary artery disease **(Figure 1-3)**. Angina is a warning sign of an impending myocardial infarction, just as a transient ischemic attack (TIA) is a warning sign of an impending stroke.

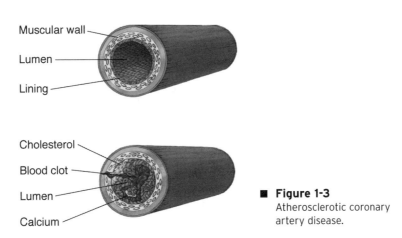

Muscular wall
Lumen
Lining

Cholesterol
Blood clot
Lumen
Calcium

■ **Figure 1-3**
Atherosclerotic coronary artery disease.

When myocardial oxygen demand increases (eg, exertion, stress), the narrowed coronary arteries are not able to supply the heart with adequate oxygenated blood flow to accommodate the increased demand, and chest pain develops (supply-demand mismatch). Once the catalyst that caused the increased oxygen demand is removed, and/or a drug such as nitroglycerin that dilates the coronary arteries is administered, the pain subsides.

Unstable angina (preinfarction angina) indicates significant occlusion of a coronary artery and occurs during nonexertional activities, or when the myocardium is otherwise in a low oxygen demand state, such as when the patient sleeps. In cases of unstable angina, the patient will describe a notable change in their typical angina pattern. Nitroglycerin may or may not be effective in relieving chest pain associated with unstable angina.

Acute myocardial infarction (AMI) occurs when a portion of the myocardium dies (undergoes necrosis), and is secondary to atherosclerotic plaque rupture, leading to a complete or near complete occlusion of a coronary artery **(Figure 1-4)**. Because the occluded artery is unable to dilate, nitroglycerin is typically ineffective in relieving the patient's chest pain.

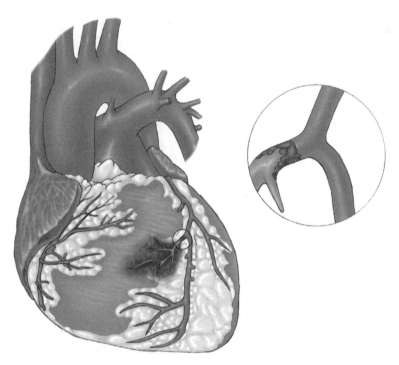

■ **Figure 1-4** Acute myocardial infarction.

The potential complications associated with acute myocardial infarction include cardiac arrest (sudden death), which occurs in up to 40% of cases, congestive heart failure, and cardiogenic shock. Although less common, ventricular rupture can occur.

4. Are the patient's vital signs and SAMPLE history consistent with your field impression?

The patient's vital signs are stable at present; however, by no means does this rule out ACS. Frequent monitoring of the patient's vital signs is important, as infarctions of the inferior myocardial wall can result in bradycardia, heart block, and hypotension.

Several findings in the SAMPLE history reinforce a field impression of ACS. First, his medical history of hypertension and angina pectoris clearly puts him in a high-risk category. Secondly, the patient's chest pressure began without exertion. And finally, both his medications are used to treat cardiovascular conditions.

■ **Atenolol (Tenormin)** is a beta-adrenergic antagonist (beta-blocker) used in the treatment of hypertension. It predominantly blocks $beta_1$-receptors, which regulate cardiac activity, thus decreasing myocardial contractility and heart rate.

■ **Nitroglycerin (NTG)** is a nitrate used in the treatment of angina pectoris. NTG relaxes the smooth muscles of the vasculature (vasodilation), thus resulting in the systemic pooling of venous blood. As a result of venous pooling, the volume of blood returned to the right atrium (preload) and systemic vascular resistance (afterload) are both decreased. The net effect of NTG is decreased cardiac workload (decreased preload and afterload) and increased myocardial oxygen supply (coronary artery dilation).

5. What specific treatment is required for this patient's condition?

- **Morphine sulfate 2 to 4 mg via slow IV push**
  - Morphine is indicated when three doses of nitroglycerin fail to completely relieve the patient's chest pain or pressure.
  - Administration of 2 to 4 mg of morphine over 1 to 5 minutes is indicated, which may be repeated every 5 to 30 minutes as needed. Morphine dosing should not exceed a maximum of 10 mg in the field unless you are directed to do so by medical control.
  - The physiologic effects of morphine include vascular smooth-muscle relaxation, which causes vasodilation and systemic venous pooling. The result is a decrease in right atrial blood return (preload) and decreased systemic vascular resistance (afterload). The narcotic analgesic effects of morphine relieve pain and anxiety, both of which are important treatments in the patient with an ACS. Morphine also suppresses sympathetic nervous system discharge, thereby lowering the patient's blood pressure and heart rate.
  - Morphine is a potent narcotic; therefore, you must closely monitor the patient for signs of central nervous system depression, such as an altered mental status, bradycardia, hypotension, and hypoventilation. If any of these effects are observed, 0.4 to 2.0 mg of naloxone hydrochloride (Narcan) should be administered via intravenous or intramuscular injection. Narcan is a narcotic antagonist that binds to opiate receptor sites in the body, thus reversing the deleterious narcotic effects.

6. Is further treatment required for this patient?

The patient is still having chest pain, although to a lesser degree. Because his blood pressure is adequate (116/74 mm Hg), you should administer another 2 to 4 mg of morphine.

Remember to monitor the patient closely for signs of central nervous system depression, such as hypotension, bradycardia, and hypoventilation, and be prepared to administer naloxone.

7. Are there any special considerations for this patient?

The risk for cardiac arrest is highest within the first hour following the onset of an ACS. Close monitoring of this patient for warning signs of impending arrest (eg, cardiac dysrhythmias) is critical.

This patient is a potential candidate for fibrinolytic (thrombolytic) therapy; therefore, you should conduct a field screening to determine his eligibility for this very important treatment. Although fibrinolytic therapy is not commonly initiated in the field, the information you obtain regarding the patient's eligibility or ineligibility will be valuable to the emergency department physician.

Numerous fibrinolytic agents are on the market **(Table 1-5)**. Their physiologic effects and indications are essentially the same.

Table 1-5 Common Fibrinolytic Agents

Alteplase, recombinant (tPA)
Anistreplase (Eminase)
Reteplase (Retavase)
Streptokinase (Streptase)
Tenecteplase (TNKase)

Fibrinolytic, or thrombolytic, therapy is used to treat patients with acute myocardial infarction and acute ischemic stroke. Fibrinolytic agents work by converting plasminogen to plasmin, the central enzyme of the physiologic fibrinolytic system. Plasmin in turn digests fibrin, the active component of a thrombus through a process called fibrinolysis. As a result of fibrinolysis, blood flow is reestablished to areas distal to the now unobstructed coronary artery, or in the case of acute ischemic stroke, cerebral artery. The indications, or inclusion criteria, for fibrinolytic therapy are summarized in **Table 1-6**.

Table 1-6 Inclusion Criteria for Fibrinolytic Therapy

Signs and symptoms of acute myocardial infarction and:
- ST-segment elevation that is 1 mm or greater in 2 or more contiguous leads
- New or presumably new left bundle-branch block
  - *Only* a 12-lead ECG can qualify these findings.
- Time of onset of symptoms is 12 hours or less.

Due to the interaction of fibrinolytic medications with the body's hematologic system, very strict criteria must be met before the patient can qualify as a candidate for therapy. In the field, paramedics must carefully screen the patient to ensure that they answer "no" to *all* of the exclusion criteria **(Table 1-7)**. If given to the wrong patient, fibrinolytics can be lethal.

Table 1-7 Exclusion Criteria for Fibrinolytic Therapy

Active internal bleeding within the past 21 days (excluding menses)
History of a cerebrovascular, intracranial, or intraspinal event within the previous three months • Stroke • Arteriovenous (AV) malformation • Neoplasm (tumor) • Aneurysm • Recent trauma or surgery
Major surgery or serious trauma within the past 14 days
Aortic dissection
Severe, uncontrolled hypertension
Known bleeding diathesis (eg, hemophilia)
Prolonged CPR with evidence of thoracic trauma
Lumbar puncture (spinal tap) within the previous 7 days
Recent arterial puncture at a noncompressible site

Summary

When managing a patient with an ACS, you should recall the mnemonic, "MONA," which stands for **m**orphine, **o**xygen, **n**itroglycerin, and **a**spirin. *Although this mnemonic does not represent the most appropriate order of treatment, it is a useful tool to help recall the appropriate management.* The correct order of medications is oxygen, aspirin, nitroglycerin, and morphine, which, when given to a patient with an ACS, focuses on decreasing myocardial oxygen demand and consumption, increasing myocardial oxygen supply, and relieving pain and anxiety.

Because the risk for cardiac arrest is greatest within the first hour following the onset of an ACS, continuous monitoring for the development of cardiac dysrhythmias is critical.

If your EMS system has the capability to obtain a 12-lead ECG tracing, you should do so. Additionally, you should screen the patient as a potential candidate for fibrinolytic medications. This information will prove useful to the emergency department physician and will decrease the "door-to-drug" time. Remember, as time progresses without treatment, permanent damage to the myocardium (heart muscle) is occurring, thus reminding us of the adage, "time is muscle."

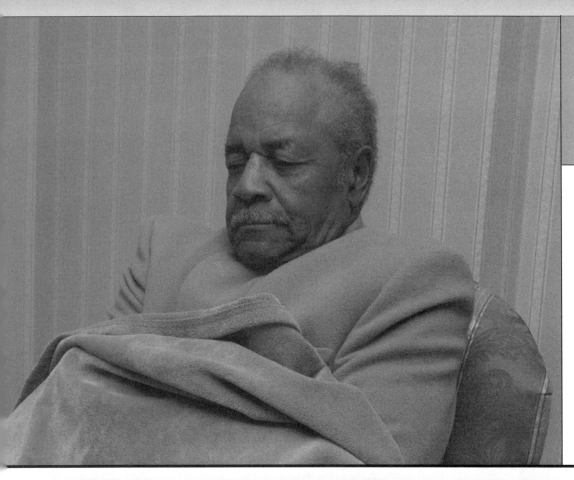

2

68-Year-Old Male with Difficulty Breathing

At 6:45 am, you receive a call to an assisted-living center at 1402 Donaldson Ave for a 68-year-old male with breathing difficulty. Your response time to the scene is approximately 5 to 7 minutes. First responders arrive shortly before you and your partner.

You arrive at the scene at 6:51 am. As you enter the patient's room, you find him sitting in a chair with a blanket up to his waist. He is in obvious respiratory distress and is noticeably pale and diaphoretic. You perform an initial assessment **(Table 2-1)** as an attendant in the assisted-living center retrieves the patient's medical records.

Table 2-1 Initial Assessment

Level of Consciousness	Responds minimally when spoken to
Chief Complaint	Difficulty breathing, altered mental status
Airway and Breathing	Respirations are rapid and profoundly labored; blood-tinged secretions are flowing from his mouth
Circulation	Radial pulses are absent; carotid pulse is rapid, weak, and irregular; skin is cool, pale, and diaphoretic

1. What initial management is indicated for this patient?

_____

_____

_____

_____

After moving the patient to the floor, your partner and a first responder begin managing the patient's airway. Meanwhile, you perform a focused history and physical examination **(Table 2-2)**. The attendant, who has returned with the patient's medical records, provides you with the information you need.

Table 2-2 Focused History and Physical Examination

Onset	"We first noticed his condition about 6 hours ago, and then it suddenly worsened."
Associated Symptoms	"He complained of chest pain yesterday, but refused to allow us to call an ambulance."
Evidence of Trauma	None
Interventions Prior to EMS Arrival	"We moved him from his bed to the chair, where we thought he would be more comfortable."
Seizures	"I haven't seen any seizures."
Fever	"No, he has not been running a fever."
Chest Exam	Intercostal retractions, sporadic chest wall movement
Breath Sounds	Coarse rhonchi are audible in all lung fields without a stethoscope.
Blood Glucose	140 mg/dL
Pupils	Dilated and slow to react

A cardiac monitor is attached and a 6-second rhythm strip is obtained **(Figure 2-1)**. You assess the cardiac rhythm as your partner and the first responder continue to manage the patient's airway.

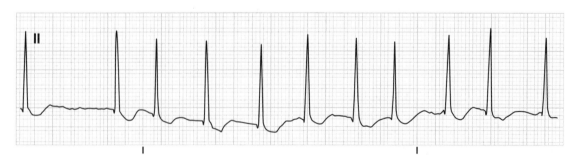

■ **Figure 2-1** Your patient's cardiac rhythm.

2. What is your interpretation of this cardiac rhythm?

_____

_____

_____

_____

Your partner advises you that the patient is now continuously producing blood-tinged secretions and his respirations are deteriorating. A first responder inserts a nasopharyngeal airway and preoxygenates the patient with a bag-valve-mask (BVM) device as your partner prepares to perform endotracheal (ET) intubation. You obtain baseline vital signs and a SAMPLE history **(Table 2-3)**. You retrieve the patient's medical history information from his medical records.

Table 2-3 Baseline Vital Signs and SAMPLE History

Blood Pressure	78/48 mm Hg
Pulse	100 beats/min, irregular and thready
Respirations	Ventilated with a BVM device at a rate of 15 breaths/min
Oxygen Saturation	94% (ventilated with 100% oxygen)
Signs and Symptoms	Altered mental status, hypotension, and pulmonary edema
Allergies	Meperidine hydrochloride (Demerol) and promethazine hydrochloride (Phenergan)
Medications	Digoxin (Lanoxin), furosemide (Lasix), potassium chloride (K-Dur), enalapril maleate (Vasotec), and warfarin sodium (Coumadin)
Pertinent Past History	Congestive heart failure, hypertension
Last Oral Intake	The patient has refused to eat for the past 2 days.
Events Leading to Present Illness	Complained of chest pain yesterday

3. What is your field impression of this patient?

_____

_____

_____

_____

4. Are the patient's vital signs and SAMPLE history consistent with your field impression?

_____

_____

_____

Knowing that you are still facing a 15-minute transport time to the closest hospital, you ask one of the first responders to retrieve the stretcher from the ambulance. Meanwhile, you attempt to start an IV of normal saline. After three attempts, you manage to secure the IV with an 18-gauge catheter. The flow rate is set to keep the vein open, at least for the time being.

5. What specific treatment is required for this patient's condition?

_____

_____

_____

The appropriate medication infusion has been initiated and the patient has been successfully intubated. The patient is placed onto the awaiting stretcher and loaded into the ambulance. You ask a first responder to drive so your partner can assist you with the patient in the back. En route, you place the patient on an automatic transport ventilator (ATV), perform an ongoing assessment **(Table 2-4)**, and then call your radio report in to the receiving hospital.

Table 2-4 Ongoing Assessment

Level of Consciousness	Improved, yet not resisting the ET tube
Airway and Breathing	Intubated and ventilated at a rate of 15 breaths/min; thick secretions present in the ET tube
Oxygen Saturation	89% (ventilated with 100% oxygen)
Blood Pressure	90 mm Hg systolic (by palpation)
Pulse	108 beats/min and irregular; weakly palpable at the radial site
Breath Sounds	Scattered rhonchi bilaterally

6. Is further treatment required for this patient?

_____

_____

_____

_____

7. Are there any special considerations for this patient?

_____

_____

_____

_____

The patient is delivered to the hospital and you give your verbal report to the charge nurse. The patient is admitted to the coronary intensive care unit after further assessment and treatment in the emergency department. Despite aggressive in-hospital care, the patient died the following day.

CASE STUDY ANSWERS AND SUMMARY

1. What initial management is indicated for this patient?

■ Positive pressure ventilation (BVM device or pocket mask device)
- The patient's respirations are severely labored and are not producing adequate tidal volume for effective oxygenation.
- In the semiconscious patient, or a patient with an intact gag reflex, a nasopharyngeal airway should be inserted to assist in maintaining airway patency.

■ Oropharyngeal suctioning
- The blood-tinged secretions must be suctioned from the patient's mouth, or they will be aspirated into the lungs, further impairing oxygenation and ventilation.
- Limit oropharyngeal suctioning to 15 seconds per attempt.

This patient's inadequate breathing and oral secretions must be managed simultaneously by suctioning the oropharynx for 15 seconds and then ventilating the patient for 2 minutes. This alternating pattern of suctioning and ventilating should continue until all secretions are cleared from the airway or the patient has been endotracheally intubated.

2. What is your interpretation of this cardiac rhythm?

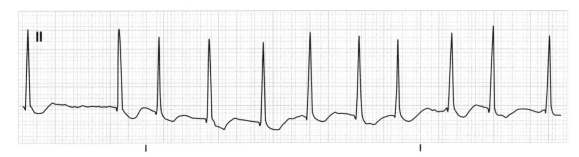

■ **Figure 2-2** Your patient's cardiac rhythm.

This cardiac rhythm **(Figure 2-2)** is irregularly irregular, has no discernable P waves, and has a ventricular rate of approximately 110 beats/min. You should easily be able to interpret this rhythm as *atrial fibrillation*. Since atrial fibrillation is an irregularly irregular rhythm, it has an irregularly irregular rate. This patient's atrial fibrillation is not much greater than 100 beats/min and is probably not the cause of his symptoms, but rather a manifestation of underlying congestive heart failure (CHF). Atrial fibrillation is commonly seen in patients with pulmonary problems that cause back pressure on the right side of the heart, such as CHF and chronic obstructive pulmonary disease (COPD).

3. What is your field impression of this patient?

This patient is clearly in shock (hypoperfusion). On the basis of your assessment findings, you should conclude that pump failure is the primary cause. Therefore, *cardiogenic shock* is the most plausible field impression. Several findings suggest a cardiogenic etiology:

■ **History of recent chest pain:** This patient was, in all likelihood, experiencing an acute myocardial infarction. However, if you recall, he refused to allow the attendant to call EMS.

■ **Blood-tinged sputum production:** This is a classic finding in severe left-sided heart failure, a common precursor to cardiogenic shock, and is the result of blood backing up in the lungs.

- **Atrial fibrillation:** Atrial dilation occurs with left-sided heart failure, often causing atrial fibrillation.

Unfortunately, cardiogenic shock has a high mortality rate of approximately 70% to 80%. It occurs when significant damage to the heart (acute or progressive) renders it unable to effectively pump blood throughout the body to meet its metabolic needs. Common causes of cardiogenic shock include acute myocardial infarction, in which a significant portion ($\geq 40\%$) of the left ventricle is destroyed; cardiomyopathy (progressive weakening of the myocardium); hypertension; and end-stage left-sided congestive heart failure.

4. Are the patient's vital signs and SAMPLE history consistent with your field impression?

This patient's vital signs only reinforce what you already know—that he is in shock! To make matters worse, his hypotension indicates a state of decompensated shock.

The entire SAMPLE history should confirm your field impression of cardiogenic shock. His cardiac history and recent chest pain make this a classic case. In addition, all of his medications are used to treat congestive heart failure, a common precursor to cardiogenic shock.

- **Digoxin (Lanoxin)** is used in the treatment of mild to moderate congestive heart failure as well as for ventricular rate control of atrial fibrillation or atrial flutter. Lanoxin increases stroke volume secondary to increased myocardial contractility (positive inotropy), thus relieving pulmonary congestion caused by left-sided heart failure.
- **Furosemide (Lasix)** is a loop diuretic used in the treatment of left-sided heart failure. Lasix inhibits sodium and chloride reabsorption in the proximal and distal tubules as well as the ascending loop of Henle in the kidneys, which results in the excretion of sodium and chloride, and, to a lesser degree, potassium and bicarbonate.
- **Potassium chloride (K-Dur)** is a potassium supplement usually prescribed concomitantly with diuretic drugs. Because diuretics promote excretion of water from the body, electrolytes such as potassium are lost as well.
- **Enalapril maleate (Vasotec)** is an angiotensin-converting enzyme (ACE) inhibitor used to treat hypertension and symptomatic CHF. ACE inhibitors suppress the renin-angiotensin-aldosterone system, thus resulting in decreased plasma levels of angiotensin II and aldosterone, both of which are potent vasoconstrictors. ACE inhibitors are usually prescribed concomitantly with diuretics in the management of CHF.
- **Warfarin sodium (Coumadin)** is an anticoagulant commonly used to treat patients with chronic atrial fibrillation. Because the atria are fibrillating, blood has a tendency to stagnate in the atria, which can result in the formation of microemboli. These microemboli may be ejected from the heart and obstruct a distant artery (eg, coronary, pulmonary, cerebral).

5. What specific treatment is required for this patient's condition?

- Dopamine, 5 to 20 µg/kg/min via IV infusion
  - This patient needs blood pressure support! You should administer medications aimed at increasing myocardial contractility (positive inotrope), which will not only improve systemic perfusion but ameliorate the pulmonary edema and improve oxygenation as well. Dopamine (Intropin) is indicated for patients with nonhypovolemic hypotension (eg, cardiogenic or neurogenic shock).
  - The dosing range for dopamine is 5 to 20 µg/kg/min, with varying physiologic effects observed at different dosing levels.

- **5 to 10 μg/kg/min (cardiac dose):** The beta effects of the dopamine dominate in this dosing range, with increases in contractility and a mild increase in heart rate. *This is the recommended dosing range for patients with cardiogenic shock.* Start the infusion at 5 μg/kg/min and titrate the infusion upward until the desired effects are achieved (eg, increased blood pressure, improved perfusion).
- **10 to 20 μg/kg/min (vasopressor dose):** Doses of greater than 10 μg/kg/min produce an alpha-adrenergic effect, thus resulting in systemic vasoconstriction. This dosing range is indicated when an emergent increase in blood pressure is required in order to prevent imminent cardiac arrest (eg, unconscious patients with a weak pulse and no obtainable blood pressure).

You may consider administering a bolus of up to 500 mL of normal saline to rule out hypovolemia prior to administering dopamine; however, extreme caution must be exercised, as excess fluids may exacerbate the patient's pulmonary edema. Consult medical direction or follow locally established protocols regarding the administration of fluid boluses in patients with cardiogenic shock and pulmonary edema.

6. Is further treatment required for this patient?

When compared with earlier assessment findings, this patient's hemodynamic status has improved (eg, improved level of consciousness, increased blood pressure). However, his oxygen saturation of 89% still suggests hypoxia. This is likely the result of the thick secretions in the ET tube, which are interfering with effective ventilation and oxygenation. Further treatment at this point should include tracheal suctioning, which should be limited to 10 seconds per attempt. Reattach the automatic ventilator for 2 to 3 minutes in-between suctioning attempts. This intervention will likely improve his oxygen saturation.

7. Are there any special considerations for this patient?

This patient needs close, continuous monitoring. Be especially observant for hypoxia-induced cardiac dysrhythmias. Should the ventricular rate of his atrial fibrillation become too fast (> 150 beats/min), pharmacological or electrical interventions may be necessary. In addition, tracheal suctioning may need to be repeated in order to maintain effective oxygenation and ventilation.

Summary

Cardiogenic shock is a condition caused by failure of the heart to effectively pump blood throughout the body. As a result, metabolic needs of the body are not met and shock (hypoperfusion) occurs.

Cardiogenic shock can occur acutely or over a period of time. Common causes include acute myocardial infarction, cardiomyopathy, hypertension, and end-stage CHF. Because of its high mortality rate of 70% to 80%, most patients with cardiogenic shock do not survive, even with aggressive prehospital and in-hospital treatment.

Managing a patient with cardiogenic shock should focus on maintaining a patent airway and supporting ventilation and circulation. Inotropic agents such as dopamine are used in order to increase myocardial contractility, which may improve blood pressure and systemic perfusion. Per medical control, a brief trial of IV fluid may be given prior to administering dopamine. Inotropic support is only a temporary measure until more definitive care can be provided at the hospital.

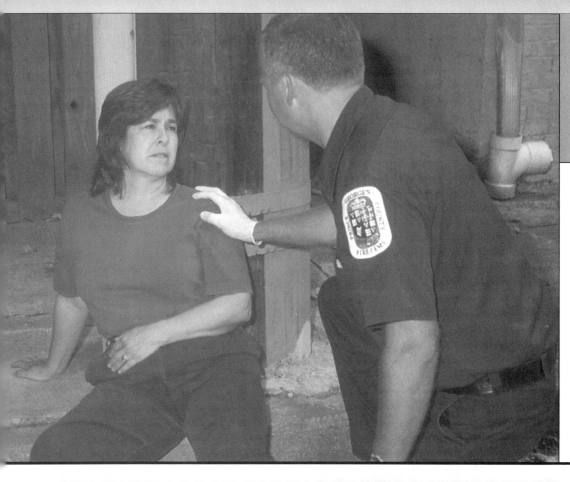

3

45-Year-Old Female with Severe Headache

At 9:44 am, you are dispatched to the 1600 block of North Main St for a 45-year-old female with a severe headache. The patient and her husband were inspecting repair work on their home and the husband called 9-1-1 on his cell phone. Your response time to the scene is approximately 5 minutes.

You arrive at the scene at 9:50 am, where you find the patient, who appears confused and disoriented, sitting on the sidewalk. You introduce yourself to the patient, and begin an initial assessment **(Table 3-1)**.

Table 3-1 Initial Assessment

Level of Consciousness	Confused and disoriented
Chief Complaint	"My head is killing me!"
Airway and Breathing	Airway is patent; respirations are normal
Circulation	Pulse is regular and bounding, rate appears normal, skin is flushed and warm

1. What initial management is indicated for this patient?

_____

_____

_____

_____

As your partner is performing the required initial management, the patient's husband tells you that his wife has high blood pressure and depression, and takes medications for both conditions.

Your partner attaches the ECG leads to the patient, as you perform a focused history and physical examination **(Table 3-2)**. The patient's husband provides you with the information you need.

Table 3-2 Focused History and Physical Examination

Description of the Episode	"She had a headache when she awoke this morning."
Onset	"I don't know exactly when the headache began."
Duration	"She has had this headache since she woke up."
Associated Symptoms	"She complained of nausea and double vision."
Evidence of Trauma	None
Interventions Prior to EMS Arrival	None
Seizures	"She has not had any seizures."
Fever	The patient is afebrile.
Blood Glucose	130 mg/dL

You ask the patient when she last took her blood pressure medication. Still confused and disoriented, she tells you that she cannot recall. Your partner hands you the patient's cardiac rhythm strip **(Figure 3-1)**.

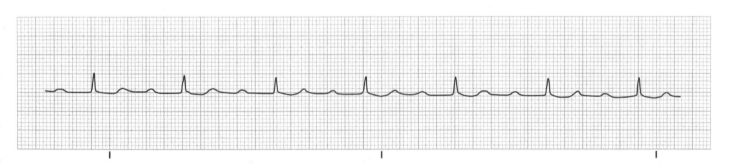

■ **Figure 3-1** Your patient's cardiac rhythm.

2. What is your interpretation of this cardiac rhythm?

_____

_____

_____

_____

The patient complains that the sun is making her headache worse, so you move her into the ambulance and dim the lights. As your partner establishes an IV of normal saline, you obtain baseline vital signs and a SAMPLE history **(Table 3-3)**.

Table 3-3 Baseline Vital Signs and SAMPLE History

Blood Pressure	210/170 mm Hg
Pulse	64 beats/min, regular and bounding
Respirations	16 breaths/min and unlabored
Oxygen Saturation	98% (on 100% oxygen)
Signs and Symptoms	Confusion, nausea, diplopia and photophobia, headache, and hypertension
Allergies	"I am allergic to Novocain."
Medications	"I take prazosin, Diuril, and Luvox."
Pertinent Past History	"I have high blood pressure, and am always depressed."
Last Oral Intake	"I can't remember when I last ate."
Events Leading to Present Illness	"I woke up this morning with this headache, which is the worst headache that I have ever had."

3. What is your field impression of this patient?

_____

_____

_____

_____

4. Are the patient's vital signs and SAMPLE history consistent with your field impression?

_____

_____

_____

_____

When you realize that the patient clearly does not need IV fluids, you set the IV line at a keep-vein-open rate. Since the closest hospital is approximately 20 miles away, you decide to transport the patient at once, while performing further interventions en route.

5. What specific treatment is required for this patient's condition?

_____

_____

_____

_____

Following your next intervention, you reassess the patient's blood pressure and note that it is 170/110 mm Hg. The patient, who is still complaining of a severe headache, appears less confused and disoriented. You complete your ongoing assessment **(Table 3-4)** and then notify the receiving hospital of your impending arrival.

Table 3-4 Ongoing Assessment

Level of Consciousness	Conscious, less confused and disoriented
Airway and Breathing	16 breaths/min and unlabored
Oxygen Saturation	98% (on 100% oxygen)
Blood Pressure	168/106 mm Hg
Pulse	60 beats/min and regular, less bounding

6. Is further treatment required for this patient?

_____

_____

_____

_____

7. Are there any special considerations for this patient?

_____

_____

_____

_____

The patient's condition continues to improve with your treatment. She is delivered to the emergency department, where her blood pressure is treated definitively.

A CT scan of her head shows no abnormalities. She is admitted to the medical intensive care unit with a diagnosis of acute hypertensive encephalopathy, and is discharged home 1 week later without neurologic deficit.

CASE STUDY ANSWERS AND SUMMARY

1. What initial management is indicated for this patient?

■ 100% oxygen via nonrebreathing mask
- This patient's respirations are adequate (normal rate and depth); therefore, she is not in need of positive pressure ventilatory support at this time.
- Patients with *any* alteration in mental status should be assumed to be suffering from cerebral hypoxia and should receive 100% supplemental oxygen as soon as possible.

2. What is your interpretation of this cardiac rhythm?

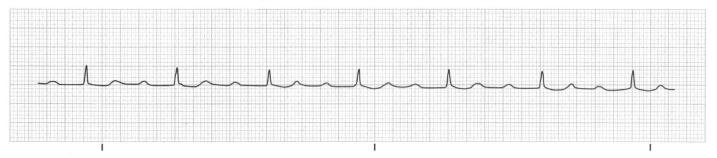

■ **Figure 3-2** Your patient's cardiac rhythm.

The characteristics of this cardiac rhythm **(Figure 3-2)** are consistent with *first-degree atrioventricular (AV) block*. The rhythm is regular, has a rate of approximately 60 beats/min, and has monomorphic P waves, all of which are consistently followed by narrow QRS complexes, and a PR interval greater than 0.20 seconds (0.40 seconds, to be exact).

First-degree AV block is typically a benign cardiac rhythm. It is characterized by a prolongation of the PR interval (> 0.20 seconds), which represents an abnormal delay at the AV junction. The normal PR interval ranges from 0.12 to 0.20 seconds.

Treatment for first-degree AV block is typically not required unless accompanied by symptomatic bradycardia. It is doubtful that this cardiac rhythm is related to this patient's signs and symptoms.

3. What is your field impression of this patient?

The first thing to note is the patient's extremely elevated blood pressure—210/170 mm Hg—which clearly indicates a hypertensive emergency. Furthermore, the following assessment findings support a field impression of *acute hypertensive encephalopathy*:

■ Disorientation

■ Severe headache

■ Nausea

■ Diplopia (double vision) and photophobia (light sensitivity)

Hypertensive encephalopathy is a life-threatening complication of severe hypertension, in which the diastolic blood pressure is 140 mm Hg or greater. If the condition is left untreated, irreversible damage to the heart, kidneys, or brain can result within a matter of a few hours.

Signs and symptoms of acute hypertensive encephalopathy include severe headache, nausea and vomiting, visual disturbances, and confusion. In severe cases, paralysis, coma, and seizures may occur.

Although conditions such as intracranial hemorrhage and pheochromocytoma (an adrenal tumor that produces epinephrine) can cause hypertensive encephalopathy, it is most commonly the result of noncompliance with antihypertensive medications in a patient with an established history of hypertension.

4. Are the patient's vital signs and SAMPLE history consistent with your field impression?

The patient's diastolic blood pressure (≥ 140 mm Hg) is consistent with a hypertensive crisis. Her respiratory and pulse rates are within normal limits; however, her pulse is bounding, which is common when the blood pressure is excessively elevated.

Any time a patient tells you that he or she is having the worst headache of their life, you should be concerned. That information alone will usually ensure that a computed tomographic (CT) scan of the head is performed at the hospital.

The patient's history of hypertension clearly predisposes her to hypertensive crisis, and her antihypertensive medications reinforce her history.

- **Prazosin (Minipress)** is a selective alpha-adrenergic blocker used to treat hypertension. Prazosin dilates arterioles and veins, thereby decreasing total peripheral vascular resistance and decreasing diastolic blood pressure more so than systolic blood pressure. Unlike beta-blocking drugs, prazosin does not cause a decrease in heart rate or cardiac output.

- **Chlorothiazide (Diuril)** is a thiazide diuretic drug commonly prescribed in combination with alpha- or beta-blocking drugs in the treatment of hypertension. Thiazides promote diuresis by decreasing the rate at which sodium and chloride are reabsorbed in the distal renal tubules in the kidney. This effect promotes the excretion of additional water from the body. Thiazides also have an antihypertensive effect, which is attributed to direct dilation of the arterioles as well as a reduction in the total fluid volume of the body.

5. What specific treatment is required for this patient's condition?

The goal in treating a hypertensive emergency involves a *rapid, yet controlled* lowering of the patient's blood pressure. If the blood pressure is lowered too fast, infarction of the heart, brain, or kidneys can occur.

In most circumstances, pharmacological therapy for hypertensive encephalopathy is initiated in the controlled setting of a hospital; however, if transport to the hospital is lengthy, or in severe cases (eg, when the patient is unconscious), medical control may order one of the following medications:

- Labetalol (Trandate, Normodyne)
  - 20 mg via slow IV push administered over 2 minutes
  - May repeat at 40 to 80 mg every 10 minutes until the desired effect is achieved or a total dose of 300 mg has been administered

- Nitroglycerin (Nitro-Bid, Tridil, Isordil, NTG)
  - Start the IV infusion at 10 µg/min and titrate to the desired effect. Do not exceed 20 µg/min.
  - Must predilute in D_5W, place in a glass bottle, and use an infusion pump

- Nitroprusside sodium (Nipride)
  - Mix 50 or 100 mg in 250 mL of D_5W *only*.
  - Start the IV infusion at 0.10 µg/kg/min and titrate upward until the desired effect is achieved. The maximum dose is 5 µg/kg/min.
  - Place opaque material around IV bottle, use an infusion pump, and carefully monitor the patient's blood pressure

Nitroglycerin would be the most common pharmacological agent used for acute hypertensive emergencies in the field, as Labetalol and Nipride are not commonly carried on the ambulance.

Placing the patient in a comfortable position and dimming the lights in the ambulance may afford the patient some relief from her headache. The patient must be transported to the hospital immediately, while monitoring airway, breathing, and circulation en route.

6. Is further treatment required for this patient?

Although the patient is less confused and disoriented, she is still dangerously hypertensive and complaining of a severe headache. At the discretion of medical control, additional medication dosing may be required. Depending on the medication that you are administering, this may involve titrating the infusion upwards (eg, Nipride, NTG), or administering another bolus dose (eg, Labetalol).

Further treatment for this patient should be supportive, which involves continuous monitoring of her airway, breathing, and circulation, and making her as comfortable as possible.

7. Are there any special considerations for this patient?

This patient is at risk for acute hemorrhagic stroke because of her significant hypertension; therefore, you must continually monitor her signs and symptoms that would indicate stroke.

Signs of acute hemorrhagic stroke include a sudden loss of consciousness and signs of increased intracranial pressure, such as bradycardia, posturing, and irregular respirations that are either fast or slow. If signs of a hemorrhagic stroke become evident, nitroglycerin would be contraindicated and should be stopped if it is being administered. Nitroglycerin would exacerbate intracranial bleeding due to its vasodilatory effects. Preparations for endotracheal intubation should be made for definitive airway control in the event that the patient loses consciousness.

Summary

Hypertensive emergencies can pose a unique challenge for the paramedic, usually because the medications used to treat them are not available for field use (eg, Nipride, Labetalol), or protocols will not allow for the emergent lowering of the blood pressure in the prehospital setting.

The priorities of care are to identify the hypertensive emergency, take measures to support airway, breathing, and circulation, and immediately transport the patient to the hospital where the blood pressure can be rapidly lowered in a controlled environment. If the patient is unconscious or otherwise unable to protect his or her own airway, intubation should be performed.

In a conscious patient, dimming the lights in the ambulance and allowing the patient to assume a comfortable position may provide relief from the severe headache that classically accompanies a hypertensive emergency.

Hypertensive encephalopathy, if left untreated, can result in irreversible damage to the heart, kidneys, and brain. Damage to these organs may be so severe that they are no longer able to support life.

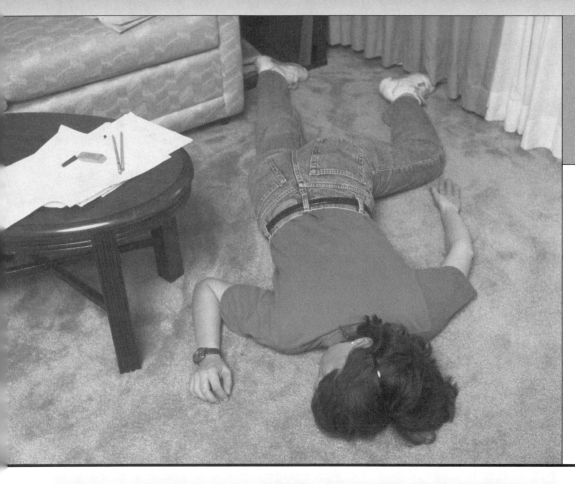

4

20-Year-Old Unconscious Female

The time is 4:45 pm. You and your partner are dispatched to a private residence at 242 Elm St for an unknown emergency. Law enforcement is dispatched to secure the scene prior to your arrival. While en route, you are notified by the police officer that the scene is secure and that an unconscious young female has been found.

Upon arrival, you enter the patient's residence and find her lying in a prone position on her living room floor. There is no evidence of trauma. After rolling the patient to a supine position, you begin your initial assessment **(Table 4-1)**. Your partner opens the jump kit and prepares to manage the patient's airway.

Table 4-1 Initial Assessment

Level of Consciousness	Unconscious and unresponsive
Chief Complaint	Unconscious and unresponsive
Airway and Breathing	Snoring respirations, slow rate, and shallow depth
Circulation	Absent radial pulses; carotid pulse is rapid and regular. Skin is flushed, hot, and dry.

1. What initial management is indicated for this patient?

_____

_____

_____

_____

Your partner is providing the appropriate initial management for the patient. As you perform a rapid patient assessment **(Table 4-2)**, a police officer hands you an empty medication bottle he found in the patient's kitchen. The bottle, which is labeled imipramine, is prescribed to the patient, and was refilled 1 day ago.

Table 4-2 Rapid Assessment

Head	No signs of trauma or bleeding
Pupils	Equal, dilated, and sluggishly reactive
Neck	Normal jugular veins, no tracheal deviation, no signs of trauma
Chest	Stable to palpation, no signs of trauma, breath sounds clear and equal bilaterally
Abdomen	Soft, nondistended, no obvious trauma, no palpable masses
Pelvis	Stable to palpation, no crepitus
Extremities (Upper and Lower)	No obvious trauma; distal pulses are weakly palpable
Posterior	No signs of trauma

Your partner secures the patient's airway with an endotracheal tube as you attach a cardiac monitor and analyze her cardiac rhythm **(Figure 4-1)**. You and your partner agree that the patient requires immediate transport.

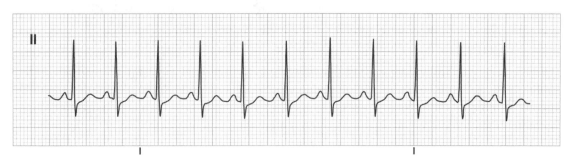

■ **Figure 4-1** Your patient's cardiac rhythm.

2. What is your interpretation of this cardiac rhythm?

_____

_____

_____

_____

You ask the police officer to retrieve the stretcher from the ambulance. As your partner continues to manage the patient's airway, you quickly obtain a set of baseline vital signs and SAMPLE history **(Table 4-3)**. Because the patient is unconscious, you are unable to obtain her medical history.

Table 4-3 Baseline Vital Signs and SAMPLE History

Blood Pressure	76/56 mm Hg
Pulse	134 beats/min, weak, and regular
Respirations	Ventilated at a rate of 20 breaths/min
Oxygen Saturation	97% (ventilated with 100% oxygen)
Signs and Symptoms	Unconscious, hypotension, tachycardia, inadequate breathing
Allergies	Unknown
Medications	Imipramine
Pertinent Past History	Unknown
Last Oral Intake	Unknown
Events Leading to Present Illness	Unknown

An IV of normal saline is established and set at a keep-vein-open rate. The police officer returns with the stretcher. The patient remains unconscious and continues receiving assisted ventilations by your partner.

3. What is your field impression of this patient?

_____

_____

_____

_____

4. Are the patient's vital signs and SAMPLE history consistent with your field impression?

_____

_____

_____

You administer up to 2 L of normal saline in an attempt to increase the patient's blood pressure. Your attempt is unsuccessful, however.

5. What specific treatment is required for this patient's condition?

_____

_____

_____

The appropriate pharmacological agent is administered via IV push. The patient is placed on the stretcher and loaded into the ambulance. En route to the hospital, you place the patient on an automatic transport ventilator (ATV) and set the ventilatory rate and tidal volume accordingly.

Shortly after completing your detailed physical examination **(Table 4-4)**, the patient experiences a grand mal seizure. You immediately tell your partner to stop the ambulance and assist you in the back with the patient.

Table 4-4 Detailed Physical Examination

Head and Face	No obvious head or facial trauma, no bleeding
Pupils	Equal, dilated, and sluggishly reactive
Airway and Breathing	Ventilated at a rate of 20 breaths/min
Neck	No obvious trauma, no jugular venous distention; trachea is midline
Chest	Chest moves symmetrically; breath sounds are clear and equal bilaterally
Abdomen	Soft and nondistended
Pelvis	Stable to palpation, no crepitation
Extremities (Upper and Lower)	Unremarkable, peripheral pulses weakly present

6. Is further treatment required for this patient?

_____

_____

_____

_____

The seizure is terminated with the appropriate medication, and transport to the hospital is resumed. Your partner radios the dispatcher, who relays your patient report to the receiving hospital. In the meantime, you perform an ongoing assessment **(Table 4-5)**.

Table 4-5 Ongoing Assessment

Level of Consciousness	Unconscious
Pupils	Equal, less dilated, more reactive
Airway and Breathing	Ventilated at a rate of 20 breaths/min
Oxygen Saturation	98% (ventilated with 100% oxygen)
Blood Pressure	90/60 mm Hg
Pulse	128 beats/min, strong and regular
Breath Sounds	Clear and equal bilaterally

7. Are there any special considerations for this patient?

_____

_____

_____

_____

The patient is delivered to the emergency department. Her vital signs have improved, yet she remains unconscious. You give your verbal report to the charge nurse. The attending physician orders blood work for chemistry analysis and a continuous infusion of sodium bicarbonate. In addition, respiratory therapists have placed the patient on a mechanical ventilator.

A 12-lead ECG is obtained, which shows a prolongation of the QT interval. The physician tells you that he is surprised the patient did not arrest in the field.

Following aggressive therapy in the emergency department, the patient is admitted to the medical intensive care unit, where she later recovered. Following discharge from the hospital, she was referred for psychiatric evaluation.

CASE STUDY ANSWERS AND SUMMARY

1. What initial management is indicated for this patient?

■ **Manual airway maneuver**
  • This patient's snoring respirations indicate partial airway obstruction by the tongue. Therefore, a manual airway maneuver is indicated.
    • Perform a head tilt–chin lift maneuver if trauma has been ruled out.
    • Perform a jaw-thrust or modified jaw-thrust maneuver if trauma is suspected or cannot be ruled out.

■ **Positive pressure ventilation (bag-valve-mask device or pocket mask device)**
  • Slow, shallow respirations will not provide adequate tidal volume needed to support effective gas exchange in the lungs.
  • Insert an oropharyngeal airway to assist in maintaining airway patency. If the patient cannot tolerate the oropharyngeal airway, insert a nasopharyngeal airway.
  • Unconscious patients are at high risk for regurgitation and aspiration. Have suction equipment readily available and be prepared to perform endotracheal intubation.

2. What is your interpretation of this cardiac rhythm?

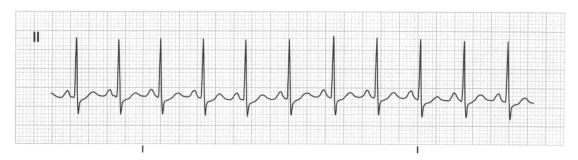

■ **Figure 4-2** Your patient's cardiac rhythm.

The patient is in *sinus tachycardia*. The rhythm **(Figure 4-2)** is regular, with a rate of approximately 130 beats/min. P waves are present, monomorphic, and consistently followed by narrow QRS complexes.

Sinus tachycardia is a manifestation of an underlying etiology. In the case of this particular patient, it indicates a sympathetic nervous system discharge and subsequent blockade of the reuptake of catecholamines (eg, epinephrine and norepinephrine), which are effects of tricyclic antidepressant drugs.

3. What is your field impression of this patient?

This patient's clinical presentation is consistent with a *tricyclic antidepressant (TCA) overdose*. Imipramine (Tofranil) is a commonly prescribed tricyclic antidepressant. Evidence that an empty bottle of medication had been refilled the day before should indicate to you that an overdose has occurred.

The following assessment findings indicate significant TCA toxicity:

■ Unconsciousness

■ Tachycardia

■ Hypotension

■ Respiratory depression

■ Hot, dry, flushed skin (indicative of fever)

When taken in excess, tricyclic antidepressants are among the most cardiotoxic drugs in medicine. The signs of toxicity result from a dangerous combination of mechanisms, all of which are related to the pharmacologic properties of tricyclics:

- Catecholamine (eg, epinephrine, norepinephrine) release and then subsequent reuptake blockage at postganglionic synapses
- Central and peripheral anticholinergic effects
- Potassium channel inhibition in the myocardium and fast sodium channel inhibition in the brain and myocardium
- Alpha-adrenergic blockade

Signs of tricyclic toxicity **(Table 4-6)** typically appear within 2 to 4 hours of significant ingestion. If the patient is asymptomatic 6 hours following ingestion, toxicity is unlikely; however, the patient should still be evaluated in the emergency department.

Table 4-6 Signs of Tricyclic Toxicity

Altered mental status, ranging from agitation and irritability to coma
Hyperpyrexia (high fever)
Mydriasis (pupillary dilation) and urinary retention secondary to the anticholinergic effects
Narrow complex tachycardias
AV heart blocks (typically preterminal)
Prolongation of the QT interval, which may lead to: • Wide QRS complexes (> 0.12 seconds)   • Wide complex tachycardias (eg, ventricular tachycardia)
Hypotension
Acidosis
Convulsions

"Three Cs and A," which stands for "Coma, Convulsions, Cardiac dysrhythmias, and Acidosis," is a helpful mnemonic to enable you to recall the signs of significant tricyclic toxicity.

4. Are the patient's vital signs and SAMPLE history consistent with your field impression?

The patient's hypotension, tachycardia, and slow, shallow respirations are all common findings in cases of significant TCA toxicity and are thus consistent with your field impression.

The empty bottle of imipramine clearly suggests an intentional overdose. The following is specific information regarding the patient's medication:

- **Imipramine (Tofranil)** was one of the first TCAs on the market. Tofranil, which is chemically related to the phenothiazine class of drugs, blocks the reuptake of norepinephrine and serotonin in the brain, thus extending its duration of action. Tofranil also has an anticholinergic effect, which depresses the parasympathetic nervous system. The therapeutic index of tricyclic drugs is very narrow, which means that even a slight increase above the therapeutic dose can result in toxicity.

5. What specific treatment is required for this patient's condition?

- 1,000-mL bolus of normal saline
  - An IV fluid bolus should be administered in an attempt to increase the patient's blood pressure.
  - If a *single* 1,000-mL bolus is unsuccessful, sodium bicarbonate should be administered immediately.
- Sodium bicarbonate 1 to 2 mEq/kg over 1 to 2 minutes.
  - The most important therapy for a patient with TCA toxicity is sodium bicarbonate-induced alkalinization. Alkalinization results in a decrease in the free, non-protein-bound form of the tricyclic molecule, and overrides the blockade of fast myocardial and cerebral sodium channels. To further achieve alkalinization, the patient should be hyperventilated (20 to 24 breaths/min) as soon as you achieve airway control. Though blood gas analysis is not available in the field, the net effect of alkalinization is to achieve a pH of 7.50 to 7.55.
  - Alkalinization with sodium bicarbonate is indicated when a TCA overdose has been confirmed (or is highly suspected) and the following signs exist:
    - QT-interval prolongation of greater than 420 ms (0.42 seconds)
    - Ventricular dysrhythmias are present (eg, V-Tach, V-Fib)
    - Hypotension that is unresponsive to a 1,000-mL bolus of normal saline

6. Is further treatment required for this patient?

In addition to ensuring adequate oxygenation and ventilation, this patient's seizure must be terminated immediately with an *anticonvulsant*. Benzodiazepines are most commonly used to terminate seizures; however, other anticonvulsants can be used as well. Commonly used medications include:

- **Lorazepam (Ativan):** 1 to 4 mg via slow IV administration over 2 to 10 minutes. This dose can be repeated in 15 to 20 minutes, to a maximum dose of 8 mg. If given intravenously, Ativan must be prediluted with an equal volume of normal saline.
- **Diazepam (Valium):** 5 mg over 2 minutes via IV push. This dose may be repeated every 10 to 15 minutes as needed, to a maximum dose of 30 mg. Diazepam is incompatible with D_5W and must be administered in an IV line of normal saline.
- **Phenytoin (Dilantin):** 1 g or 15 to 20 mg/kg via slow IV push. Do not exceed a dose of 1 g or a rate of 50 mg/min. Doses of 100 to 150 mg can be repeated in 30-minute intervals. Use an inline filter when administering Dilantin, and flush the IV line with 10 to 20 mL of normal saline, both before and after administering the drug.

Refer to your locally established protocols or contact medical control as needed, as other medications may be used in the management of seizures. The longer the seizure persists, the greater the chance of hypoxic death!

7. Are there any special considerations for this patient?

Although the patient is in a narrow complex tachycardia at present, prolongation of the QT interval, common in cases of significant TCA toxicity, could result in ventricular tachycardia, with rapid deterioration to ventricular fibrillation and cardiac arrest.

Although the normal QT interval **(Figure 4-3)** varies with factors such as the heart rate and the patient's age and sex, it should typically be less than half the duration of the R-R interval.

A 12-lead ECG should be obtained if available in the field and the QT interval carefully assessed for prolongation.

Sodium bicarbonate administration and continued hyperventilation of this patient are necessary in order to achieve alkalosis, which is the mainstay in the management of a TCA overdose.

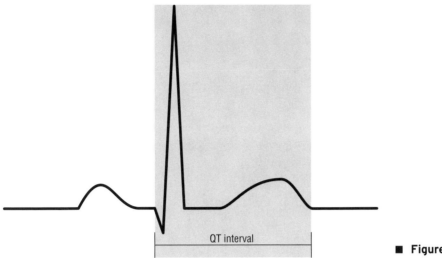
QT interval

■ **Figure 4-3** The QT interval.

Summary

Millions of Americans are prescribed TCAs by their physicians. In therapeutic doses, they are very effective in treating depression as well as other select conditions. When taken in excess, however, these drugs can be and are often deadly. Commonly prescribed tricyclics include imipramine (Tofranil), nortriptyline (Pamelor), amitriptyline (Elavil), clomipramine (Anafranil), and desipramine (Norpramin).

In cases of suspected overdose, it is critical that the paramedic identifies the substance ingested and the time it was ingested. Treatment aimed at supporting airway, breathing, and circulation, and alkalinizing the patient's blood need to be initiated immediately. Seizures are a common manifestation of significant TCA toxicity and should be managed with benzodiazepines (eg, Valium, Ativan).

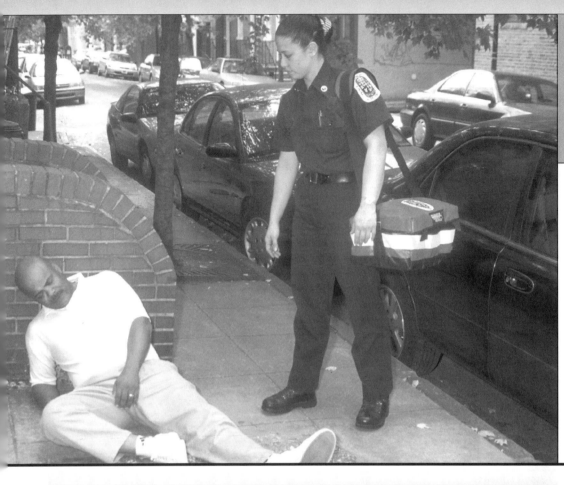

5

49-Year-Old Semiconscious Male

At 5:52 pm, you are dispatched to 9060 E Southcross Blvd for a 49-year-old man who suddenly collapsed after he and his wife returned home from dinner. Your response time to the scene is approximately 5 minutes.

You arrive at the scene at 5:56 pm, where you find the patient sitting up against a small brick wall in front of a house. He is semiconscious, and his breathing appears irregular. His wife tells you that he suddenly grabbed his head, complaining of a severe headache, and then sat down. When she tried to talk to him, he would not answer her. After ruling out trauma, you perform an initial assessment of the patient **(Table 5-1)**.

Table 5-1 Initial Assessment

Level of Consciousness	Responsive to painful stimuli only
Chief Complaint	According to his wife, a "sudden, severe headache"
Airway and Breathing	Airway is patent; respirations are rapid and irregular
Circulation	Radial pulse is slow and bounding; skin is warm and dry

1. What initial management is indicated for this patient?

_____

_____

_____

_____

As your partner performs the appropriate initial management, you conduct a focused history and physical examination **(Table 5-2)**. Because the patient is unable to communicate with you, you obtain the required information from his wife.

Table 5-2 Focused History and Physical Examination

Description of the Episode	"He grabbed his head, and then sat down. He only mumbled when I spoke to him."
Onset	"This happened suddenly."
Duration	"He has been like this since I called 9-1-1."
Associated Symptoms	"Nothing that I can recall."
Evidence of Trauma	None
Interventions Prior to EMS Arrival	"I didn't do anything other than call 9-1-1."
Seizures	"I didn't notice any seizures."
Fever	The patient is afebrile.
Pupils	4 mm bilaterally, sluggish to react
Blood Glucose	140 mg/dL
GCS	8

You attach a cardiac monitor and analyze the patient's cardiac rhythm **(Figure 5-1)**. Your partner continues ventilatory assistance, and makes preparations to intubate the patient due to his low Glasgow Coma Scale (GCS) score **(Table 5-3)**, and to more effectively protect his airway from vomiting and aspiration.

Table 5-3 Your Patient's Glasgow Coma Scale

Eye Opening	Reacts to pain (2)
Verbal Response	Incomprehensible sounds (2)
Motor Response	Withdraws from pain (4)

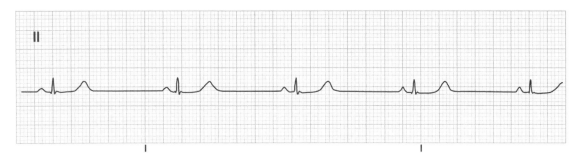

II

■ **Figure 5-1** Your patient's cardiac rhythm.

2. What is your interpretation of this cardiac rhythm?

_____

_____

_____

The patient's teeth are clenched, making intubation difficult. After initiating an IV line of normal saline, you administer 2.0 mg of midazolam (Versed), 0.04 to 0.1 mg/kg of pancuronium bromide (Pavulon), and 1.0 mg/kg of lidocaine. After these drugs are administered in a rapid sequence, the patient is successfully intubated and ventilatory support is continued. You quickly obtain baseline vital signs and a SAMPLE history **(Table 5-4)**. The patient's wife provides you with this information.

Table 5-4 Baseline Vital Signs and SAMPLE History

Blood Pressure	170/110 mm Hg
Pulse	48 beats/min and bounding
Respirations	Ventilated at a rate of 10 breaths/min
Oxygen Saturation	96% (ventilated with 100% oxygen)
GCS	Unable to obtain since the patient has been given a paralytic
Signs and Symptoms	Semiconscious, hypertension, bradycardia, and irregular breathing
Allergies	"He is allergic to codeine."
Medications	Corgard, DiaBeta
Pertinent Past History	"He has high blood pressure and non-insulin-dependent diabetes."
Last Oral Intake	"We ate dinner approximately 1 hour ago."
Events Leading to Present Illness	"He complained of a sudden, severe headache."

3. What is your field impression of this patient?

_____

_____

_____

_____

4. Are the patient's vital signs and SAMPLE history consistent with your field impression?

_____

_____

_____

_____

You quickly place the patient onto the stretcher, load him into the ambulance, and begin transport to the closest appropriate facility, which is approximately 10 miles away. The patient's wife rides in the front seat of the ambulance.

5. What specific treatment is required for this patient's condition?

_____

_____

_____

_____

En route to the hospital, you place the patient on an automatic transport ventilator (ATV), set the ventilatory rate and tidal volume accordingly, and perform an ongoing assessment **(Table 5-5)**.

Table 5-5 Ongoing Assessment

Level of Consciousness	Unconscious (paralyzed with neuromuscular blockade and sedated)
Airway and Breathing	Ventilated at a rate of 10 breaths/min
Oxygen Saturation	97% (ventilated with 100% oxygen)
Blood Pressure	162/118 mm Hg
Pulse	44 beats/min and bounding
Pupils	4 mm bilaterally, sluggishly reactive
GCS	Unable to obtain since the patient has been given a paralytic

Despite your aggressive treatment, the patient's condition deteriorates en route. Shortly before you call your report to the receiving facility, the patient experiences a grand mal seizure.

6. Is further treatment required for this patient?

The seizure is terminated pharmacologically. You reauscultate the patient's breath sounds, which remain clear and equal bilaterally. Additionally, the end-tidal CO_2 detector confirms correct tube placement. You call your radio report to the receiving hospital, and inform hospital personnel of your impending arrival.

7. Are there any special considerations for this patient?

The patient's condition is unchanged upon arrival at the hospital. After further assessment and management in the emergency department, a CT scan of the patient's head is obtained **(Figure 5-2)**, which reveals a large intracerebral hemorrhage.

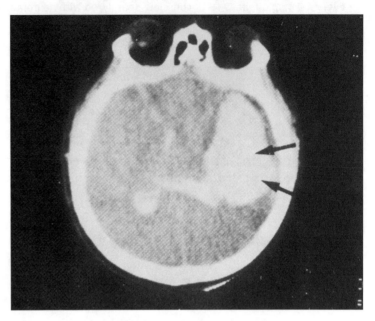

■ **Figure 5-2** Large intracerebral hemorrhage.

As the patient was being prepared for emergency surgery, cardiac arrest occurred and the patient died. Upon following up with the hospital later, you learn that the patient's brain herniated, which resulted in cardiac arrest.

1. What initial management is indicated for this patient?

- Positive pressure ventilation (bag-valve-mask device or pocket mask device)
  - The patient's rapid, irregular breaths are not providing adequate tidal volume; therefore, ventilatory support is needed to achieve effective oxygenation.
  - The appropriate ventilatory rate for this patient is 10 breaths/min.
  - Insert a nasopharyngeal airway to assist in maintaining airway patency.
  - Because the patient is semiconscious, he is at high risk for regurgitation and aspiration. Therefore, suction equipment should be readily available, and preparations for intubation should be made.

2. What is your interpretation of this cardiac rhythm?

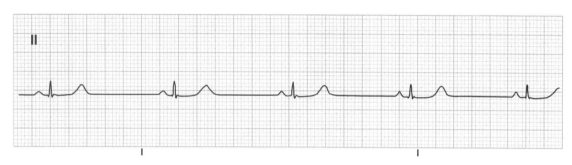

- **Figure 5-3** Your patient's cardiac rhythm.

This is a slow, narrow complex rhythm, with a ventricular rate of approximately 45 beats/min **(Figure 5-3)**. P waves are present, monomorphic, and consistently followed by narrow QRS complexes. These attributes make this rhythm a *sinus bradycardia*.

Sinus bradycardia is the result of increased parasympathetic nervous system discharge. As you will recall, the parasympathetic nervous system, also referred to as the cholinergic nervous system, is responsible for vegetative functions such as resting heart rate and blood pressure.

The chemical neurotransmitter of the parasympathetic nervous system is acetylcholine, which acts upon the vagus nerve and slows the heart rate.

Common causes of sinus bradycardia include inferior wall myocardial infarction, in which the bradycardia is commonly associated with an AV heart block, diseases of the sinus node, and increased intracranial pressure (ICP), in which the bradycardia is a reflex response to hypertension. In some patients, especially those who are well-conditioned, sinus bradycardia may be a normal finding.

3. What is your field impression of this patient?

This patient is suffering from a *hemorrhagic stroke* and is showing signs of increased ICP. Several key findings reinforce this field impression:

- Sudden, severe headache
- Rapid decline in level of consciousness
- Rapid, irregular breathing
- Sluggishly reactive pupils

A hemorrhagic stroke, which is less common than an ischemic stroke, can occur as the result of a ruptured cerebral aneurysm (weakened cerebral artery), or an arteriovenous (AV) malformation (collection of abnormal cerebral blood vessels).

Typically, aneurysms occur on the brain's surface and hemorrhage into the parenchyma (tissue) of the brain or into the subarachnoid space. Hemorrhage from an arteriovenous malformation generally originates within the parenchyma of the brain, the subarachnoid space, or both. In either circumstance, bleeding is occurring within the brain **(Figure 5-4)**, which increases ICP.

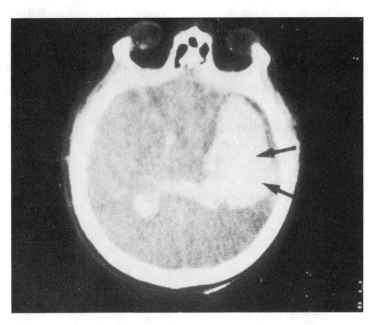

■ **Figure 5-4** Large intracerebral hemorrhage.

Hypertension is the most common precursor to hemorrhagic stroke; however, frequent use of cocaine and other sympathomimetics can also precipitate this catastrophic event secondary to a drug-induced hypertension.

The onset of hemorrhagic stroke is often acute and marked by a severe headache, followed by a rapid deterioration in level of consciousness. Because little extra space exists within the cranium, intracerebral bleeding rapidly increases ICP.

The presentation and progression of the patient's signs and symptoms are directly related to increasing ICP and follow a somewhat predictable pattern. As ICP rises, the upper portion of the brainstem is compressed, the blood pressure increases in order to maintain cerebral perfusion pressure (CPP), and a reflex bradycardia occurs in response to parasympathetic stimulation of the vagus nerve (cranial nerve X).

Abnormal respiratory patterns are seen as a result of pressure on various portions of the brainstem. Cheyne-Stokes breathing is characterized by a speeding and slowing of the patient's breathing alternating with periods of apnea and indicates pressure on the upper portion of the brainstem. Central neurogenic hyperventilation is characterized by deep, rapid respirations, and is seen with compression of the middle portion of the brainstem. Biot's (ataxic) breathing is characterized by breathing that varies in rate and depth, with periods of apnea, and indicates pressure on the lower portion of the brainstem.

The combination of hypertension, bradycardia, and abnormal breathing is referred to as Cushing's Triad, and indicates significant elevation of ICP **(Table 5-6)**.

Table 5-6 Cushing's Triad

Hypertension
Bradycardia
Abnormal respiratory patterns
• Cheyne-Stokes breathing
• Central neurogenic hyperventilation
• Biot's breathing

Other signs of increasing ICP include projectile vomiting and body temperature changes, which result from hypothalamus involvement, and decorticate (flexion) posturing in response to painful stimuli, which indicates upper brainstem compression.

ICP will eventually increase to a point where herniation (external or internal) of the brain occurs. External herniation occurs when the brainstem is forced from the cranial vault through the foramen magnum. Internal herniation occurs when the temporal lobe of the brain is forced through the tentorium incisura (opening in the dura mater). During herniation, the oculomotor nerve (cranial nerve III) is compressed, resulting in pupillary dilation on the ipsilateral (same) side of the hemorrhage. As herniation progresses, bilateral pupillary dilation, caused by compression of the contralateral (opposite) oculomotor nerve, is seen. Decerebrate (extension) posturing is also seen during late cerebral herniation.

Finally, ICP increases to the point where cerebral perfusion pressure falls below 60 mm Hg and brain cells begin to die. Hypotension and tachycardia develop, followed by cardiac arrest.

4. Are the patient's vital signs and SAMPLE history consistent with your field impression?

The patient's vital signs are consistent with Cushing's Triad, as discussed earlier. Additionally, the pulse pressure, or the difference between the systolic and diastolic blood pressure, will become widened as ICP increases.

The patient's medical history of hypertension certainly places him in a high-risk category for hemorrhagic stroke. His medical history is confirmed by the antihypertensive medication that he is taking.

■ **Nadolol (Corgard)** possesses both beta$_1$- and beta$_2$-adrenergic blocking actions. It is prescribed alone or with thiazide diuretics in the management of hypertension.

5. What specific treatment is required for this patient's condition?

■ **Endotracheal intubation**
  • Intubation will more effectively protect his airway from aspiration should vomiting occur.
  • Patients with a GCS of less than 8 should be endotracheally intubated.
  • If the patient's teeth are clenched, rapid sequence induction (RSI) will be necessary in order to facilitate intubation. Administer a sedative (eg, Ativan, Versed), followed by a neuromuscular blocker (eg, Pavulon, Norcuron). One to 1.5 mg/kg of lidocaine should also be given to minimize the increased ICP commonly associated with intubation.

- **Ensure effective ventilation**
  - Ventilate the patient at a rate of 10 breaths/min to maintain CPP.
  - Routine hyperventilation of the patient with elevated ICP should be avoided as this may cause profound cerebral vasoconstriction, resulting in decreased CPP.
  - Hyperventilate the patient at a rate of 20 breaths/min *only* if signs of cerebral herniation are present. This *may* buy the patient some time by transiently reducing ICP (at the expense of CPP) until neurosurgical interventions can be performed.
    - These ventilatory rates are recommended by the Brain Trauma Foundation (BTF).

Signs of cerebral herniation that would necessitate hyperventilation include bilaterally fixed (nonreactive) and dilated pupils, asymmetric (unequal) pupils, and decerebrate posturing or total body flaccidity.

- **IV fluid resuscitation**
  - Because he is hypertensive, fluid boluses are not indicated and will only worsen his ICP.
    - If the patient experiences hypotension (systolic BP < 90 mm Hg), isotonic crystalloid fluids should be given to maintain a systolic BP of 90 mm Hg. Hypotension in the patient with an already decreased CPP can be rapidly fatal.

Unless used to facilitate endotracheal intubation (eg, paralytics, lidocaine), pharmacological agents are typically not given in the field to patients with a hemorrhagic stroke. You should contact medical control and/or refer to locally established protocols regarding which, if any, medications are to be administered.

6. Is further treatment required for this patient?

This patient's seizure is secondary to increased ICP and must be terminated immediately with a benzodiazepine drug. One of the following medications should be administered:

- **Lorazepam (Ativan):** 1 to 4 mg via slow IV administration over 2 to 10 minutes. This dose can be repeated in 15 to 20 minutes, to a maximum dose of 8 mg. If given intravenously, Ativan must be prediluted with an equal volume of normal saline.
- **Diazepam (Valium):** 5 mg over 2 minutes via IV push. This dose may be repeated every 10 to 15 minutes as needed, to a maximum dose of 30 mg.

You must reevaluate placement of the endotracheal tube, which·may have become dislodged during the seizure. In the event that the patient becomes combative, additional sedation with midazolam (Versed) will be required. Further dosing of pancuronium bromide (Pavulon) may be necessary as well to maintain neuromuscular blockade (paralysis).

7. Are there any special considerations for this patient?

It is clear that this patient's condition is grave. Continuous monitoring is critical, specifically for signs of progressive brain herniation and cardiac dysrhythmias. Due to pressure on the brainstem and cerebral hypoxia, cardiac dysrhythmias are commonly associated with increased ICP and can lead to cardiac arrest. If this occurs, follow standard ACLS protocols to include defibrillation for ventricular fibrillation and pulseless ventricular tachycardia and epinephrine every 3 to 5 minutes.

Frequently monitor the patient's vital signs, paying particular attention to the pulse pressure. Progressive widening of the pulse pressure indicates worsening ICP and impending herniation. Maintain a ventilatory rate of 10 breaths/min unless signs of herniation are present.

Consideration should be given to this patient for potential organ harvesting, especially because his condition will likely have a poor outcome. If possible, maintain a systolic blood pressure of 90 mm Hg in order to maintain CPP and perfusion of the vital organs such as the heart, lungs, liver, kidneys, and pancreas. These organs potentially could be used to save many lives.

Summary

In contrast to the ischemic stroke, which accounts for approximately 85% of all strokes and rarely leads to death within the first hour, hemorrhagic strokes represent the remaining 15% of all strokes and can be rapidly fatal. Additionally, the signs and symptoms of hemorrhagic stroke develop abruptly, followed by rapid deterioration of the patient's condition.

Hemorrhagic strokes are commonly associated with factors such as chronic hypertension and stress or exertion. Sympathomimetic drugs, such as cocaine, can also cause a hemorrhagic stroke secondary to a rapid elevation in blood pressure, which ruptures a cerebral artery.

Management of the patient with a hemorrhagic stroke is aimed at protecting the airway, maintaining effective ventilation (not hyperventilation), maintaining a systolic blood pressure of at least 90 mm Hg with crystalloid IV fluids, and rapidly transporting the patient to the closest appropriate facility for neurosurgical intervention. Seizures should be terminated with a benzodiazepine drug (eg, Ativan, Valium).

As with patients with closed head injury, those with a hemorrhagic stroke can be difficult to intubate due to clenching of the teeth (trismus). If this occurs, rapid sequence induction (eg, sedation, neuromuscular blockade, and lidocaine) may be necessary in order to facilitate intubation.

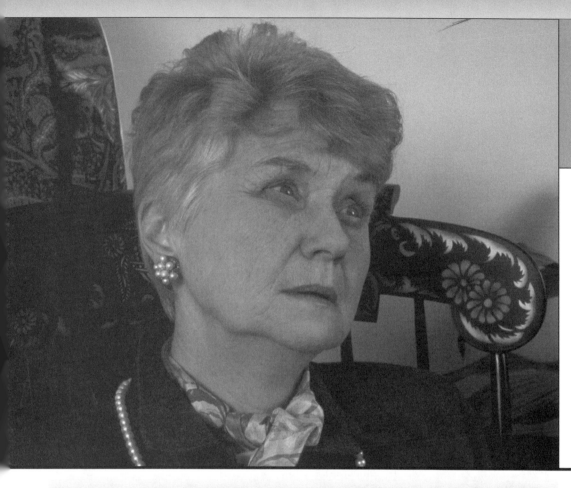

6

66-Year-Old Female Who Is Confused and Disoriented

At 9:14 am, you are dispatched to 1455 N Wagonwheel Dr. A medical alert company called 9-1-1 after a distress alarm was activated from that location. You and your partner, an EMT-I, respond to the scene, which is approximately 6 minutes away from your station.

The police arrive before you and determine that the scene is safe. When you arrive, you enter the residence and find a disoriented 66-year-old female sitting in a chair in her living room. She is obviously diaphoretic. The patient's daughter, who activated the medical alarm, gives your partner additional information as you perform an initial assessment **(Table 6-1)**.

Table 6-1 Initial Assessment

Level of Consciousness	Confused and disoriented
Chief Complaint	According to the daughter, "She is not acting right."
Airway and Breathing	Airway patent; respirations increased, with adequate tidal volume
Circulation	Weak radial pulses with normal rate; skin is diaphoretic

1. What initial management is indicated for this patient?

_____

_____

_____

_____

Your partner provides the appropriate initial management as you conduct a focused history and physical examination **(Table 6-2)**. Because the patient is confused and is unable to recall the preceding events, her daughter provides you with as much information as she can.

Table 6-2 Focused History and Physical Examination

Description of the Episode	"I called my mother, who sounded very confused and disoriented, so I came right over to see if she was alright."
Onset	"I was not present when this began."
Duration	"She has been like this for at least 30 minutes."
Associated Symptoms	"She told me that she has a headache, and vomited once this morning."
Evidence of Trauma	None
Interventions Prior to EMS Arrival	None
Seizures	"I have not witnessed any seizures."
Fever	Oral temperature is 101.9° F
Blood Glucose	48 mg/dL
Pupils	Equal and reactive to light

Noting the blood glucose level of 48 mg/dL, you ask the daughter if her mother has a history of diabetes or hypoglycemia. The daughter denies this, but says that she does have high blood pressure.

Your partner attaches the ECG leads to the patient, obtains a 6-second rhythm strip **(Figure 6-1)**, and hands it to you for interpretation.

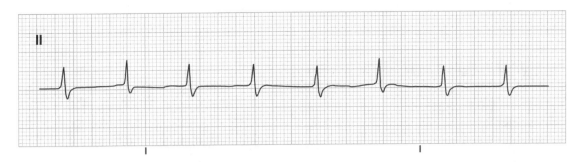

■ **Figure 6-1** Your patient's cardiac rhythm.

2. What is your interpretation of this cardiac rhythm?

_____

_____

_____

_____

Your partner initiates an IV line of normal saline and sets the flow rate to keep the vein open. In the meantime, you obtain baseline vital signs and a SAMPLE history **(Table 6-3)**. The patient's daughter provides you with the information.

Table 6-3 Baseline Vital Signs and SAMPLE History

Blood Pressure	138/78 mm Hg
Pulse	84 beats/min, weak and regular
Respirations	24 breaths/min and unlabored
Oxygen Saturation	98% (on 100% oxygen)
Signs and Symptoms	Confusion, disorientation, headache, weak pulse
Allergies	"She is allergic to penicillin and aspirin."
Medications	"She takes Levatol for her blood pressure."
Pertinent Past History	"She has high blood pressure, and had breast cancer 15 years ago."
Last Oral Intake	"When I spoke with her last evening, she had just eaten supper. I assume that this was the last time she ate."
Events Leading to Present Illness	"I called her this morning, and she sounded confused and disoriented."

3. What is your field impression of this patient?

_____

_____

_____

_____

4. Are the patient's vital signs and SAMPLE history consistent with your field impression?

_____

_____

_____

The patient's daughter requests that you transport her mother to a hospital, which is approximately 15 miles away. You explain your transport decision to the patient. She remains confused and disoriented, but agrees to transport. Your partner retrieves the stretcher from the ambulance.

5. What specific treatment is required for this patient's condition?

_____

_____

_____

Following further treatment, the patient's mental status has markedly improved. You place her onto the stretcher, load her into the ambulance, and begin transport. En route, you perform an ongoing assessment **(Table 6-4)**.

Table 6-4 Ongoing Assessment

Level of Consciousness	Conscious and alert to person, place, and time
Airway and Breathing	Respirations, 18 breaths/min and unlabored
Oxygen Saturation	99% (on 100% oxygen)
Blood Pressure	140/68 mm Hg
Pulse	86 beats/min, strong and regular
Blood Glucose	130 mg/dL
Pupils	Equal and reactive to light

6. Is further treatment required for this patient?

_____

_____

_____

_____

You call your radio report to the receiving facility and relay the patient's initial presentation and subsequent response to your treatment. Your estimated time of arrival at the hospital is 10 minutes.

7. Are there any special considerations for this patient?

_____

_____

_____

_____

The patient is delivered to the hospital in stable condition. You give your verbal report to the attending physician. Blood is drawn for lab analysis, and a chest radiograph is ordered.

The patient is admitted to the hospital for a bacterial infection and is treated with fluid hydration and antibiotics. After a 7-day stay in the hospital, she is discharged home.

CASE STUDY ANSWERS AND SUMMARY

1. What initial management is indicated for this patient?

- **100% oxygen via nonrebreathing mask**
  - Although the rate of respirations is increased, they are of adequate depth; therefore, positive pressure ventilatory support is not required at this time.
  - *Any* patient with an altered mental status should be given 100% supplemental oxygen as soon as possible.

2. What is your interpretation of this cardiac rhythm?

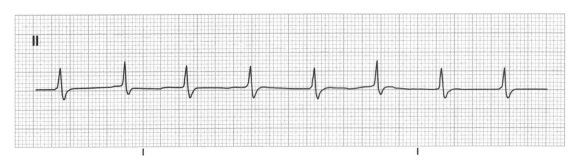

- **Figure 6-2** Your patient's cardiac rhythm.

This cardiac rhythm is regular, with a rate of approximately 85 beats/min, and has narrow QRS complexes **(Figure 6-2)**. No P waves are seen with this rhythm, however. Because of this absence and the regular rate, you should interpret this as an *accelerated junctional rhythm*.

Junctional rhythms originate from an escape pacemaker in the atrioventricular (AV) junction. Junctional rhythms are a normal response of the AV junction when the sinoatrial (SA) node fails as the primary pacemaker, or when the electrical discharge rate of the SA node falls below that of the AV junctional escape pacemaker (40 to 60 beats/min).

There are three categories of junctional rhythms: escape, accelerated, and tachycardia, with the ventricular rate determining the category. Junctional escape rhythms typically range from 40 to 60 beats/min, accelerated junctional rhythms range from 60 to 100 beats/min, and junctional tachycardia has a rate greater than 100 beats/min.

Junctional rhythms could indicate myocardial ischemia or infarction or sinus node disease. In this particular patient, no correlation appears to exist between her signs and symptoms and her cardiac rhythm.

3. What is your field impression of this patient?

Don't let the patient's absent history of diabetes or hypoglycemia fool you! This patient is indeed suffering from *hypoglycemia,* most likely secondary to an infection (she has a fever).

The following pertinent findings support a field impression of infection-induced hypoglycemia:

- **Blood glucose level of 48 mg/dL:** Normal blood glucose levels range from 80 to 120 mg/dL. Typically, patients will become symptomatic when their blood glucose levels fall below 60 mg/dL.
- **Confusion and disorientation:** The brain requires glucose just as it does oxygen. The patient with hypoglycemia therefore will present with mental status changes

identical to those of hypoxia, such as restlessness, confusion, disorientation, and combativeness.

- **Diaphoresis:** This is a common sign found in patients with hypoglycemia.
- **Documented fever:** A temperature of 101.9° F confirms the presence of an infectious process. As the body attempts to fight off an infection, a great deal of energy, which requires glucose, is expended. In children and the elderly, glucose stores are rapidly depleted.

4. Are the patient's vital signs and SAMPLE history consistent with your field impression?

The patient's increased respiratory rate is consistent with hypoglycemia. Her heart rate of 84 beats/min, lower than you would expect of the hypoglycemic patient, is most likely an effect of her Levatol, which is a beta-blocker. Patients who take beta-blockers may not respond with tachycardia to conditions that would require an increase in heart rate (eg, hypoglycemia, hypovolemia, or hypoxia).

The patient had not eaten since the previous evening. A combination of not eating and the apparent infection would clearly predispose her to hypoglycemia. Information regarding the patient's medication is as follows:

- **Penbutolol (Levatol)** is a beta-adrenergic blocker used to treat hypertension. It blocks the sympathetic nervous system's release of epinephrine and norepinephrine, which results in vasodilation, decreased myocardial contractility (negative inotropy), and lowering of the heart rate. These combined effects lower the blood pressure.

5. What specific treatment is required for this patient's condition?

- **Draw a red top tube of blood**
  - This will allow the hospital to get a pretreatment blood glucose reading as well as the patient's electrolyte levels, which may have contributed to her hypoglycemia. It should be noted that in critical patients, such as those who are unconscious, you should not delay further treatment in order to draw blood.
- **25 to 50 g (50 to 100 mL) of 50% dextrose**
  - A blood glucose reading of less than 60 mg/dL, with accompanying signs and symptoms, should be treated with 50% dextrose.
  - Give an initial bolus of 25 g (50 mL), and reassess the patient. If symptoms persist, another 25 g of dextrose may be necessary.

If IV access cannot be obtained, there are alternative treatments for patients with hypoglycemia.

- **Oral glucose (1 to 2 tubes)**
  - If the patient is conscious and alert enough to swallow, administer 1 to 2 tubes of oral glucose, and then reassess the blood glucose. The patient usually self-administers this medication.
    - Oral glucose also comes in a tablet form.
- **Glucagon 0.5 to 1.0 mg intramuscularly**
  - Glucagon is produced in the alpha cells of the pancreas. Its production results in the elevation of blood glucose levels by increasing the breakdown of glycogen, which is produced in the liver, to glucose (glycogenolysis) and stimulating glucose synthesis (gluconeogenesis).
  - Glucagon administration is effective *only* if the patient has adequate stores of glycogen in their liver. Glucagon cannot break down glycogen if it does not exist.

- Prior to administration of glucagon, reconstitute it by diluting 1 mg (white powder) in 1 mL of provided diluent. Do not dilute glucagon with normal saline. The 0.5- to 1.0-mg dose can be repeated if there is no response.
- The onset of action of glucagon ranges from 5 to 20 minutes, with the maximum effects seen 30 minutes after administration. The duration of action of glucagon ranges from 1 to 2 hours.

6. Is further treatment required for this patient?

At this point, the patient's mental status and blood glucose level have shown marked improvement. Continuing oxygen therapy and repeating a blood glucose reading would be the only interventions required at this point.

7. Are there any special considerations for this patient?

With the continued fever, this patient's immune system is fighting off an infection. As previously mentioned, this process requires energy, and energy requires glucose, which can be rapidly depleted.

You should monitor this patient's mental status and recheck her blood glucose reading. If her mental status becomes altered and her blood glucose level falls below 60 mg/dL, additional medication therapy (eg, 50% dextrose, glucagon) will be required.

Summary

A patient medical history that does not include diabetes or hypoglycemia does not automatically rule out the possibility of the patient having a low blood glucose level. Hypoglycemia, although clearly more common in the diabetic patient, is by no means exclusive to that particular patient population.

Both pediatric and geriatric patients have limited glycogen stores, which are rapidly depleted by conditions that would typically not affect other age groups. Factors such as strenuous exertion, infection, and a few missed meals could easily result in hypoglycemia.

The assessment for any patient with an altered mental status should include a blood glucose reading, whether the patient has a history of diabetes or not. If the blood glucose level is less than 60 mg/dL and the patient is symptomatic, 50% dextrose should be administered. If IV access is not possible, glucagon can be administered intramuscularly. If glucagon is not carried on your ambulance and the patient is conscious and alert enough to swallow, administer 1 to 2 tubes of oral glucose.

Further management consists of 100% supplemental oxygen therapy or positive pressure ventilatory support if the patient is breathing inadequately.

Hypoglycemia is perhaps one of the most easily treated medical emergencies. However, if not recognized and treated promptly, it can rapidly lead to death. Remember, the brain needs glucose as much as it does oxygen, and will simply cease to function in its absence.

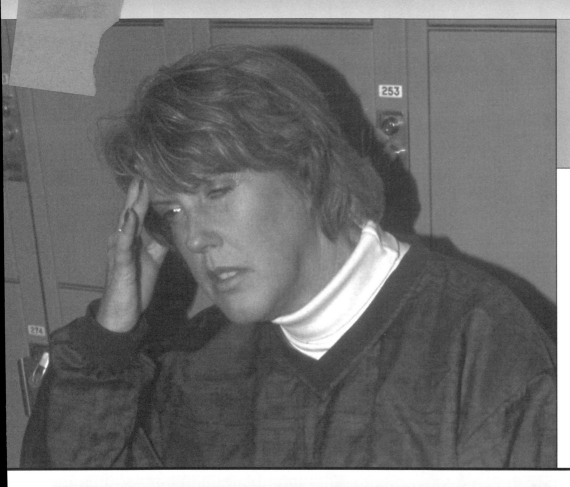

7

41-Year-Old Female with Nausea and Headache

Your unit is dispatched to a middle school at 141 E Blanco St for a 41-year-old female who is "sick." You and your partner respond to the scene, which is 3 miles from your station. The time of call is 8:10 am.

You arrive at the scene, enter the school building, and find the patient, a middle-school teacher, standing outside her classroom. Obviously disoriented, she tells you that she woke up this morning with a headache and nausea. You perform an initial assessment (Table 7-1) as your partner opens the jump kit and prepares to initiate treatment.

Table 7-1 Initial Assessment

Level of Consciousness	Disoriented
Chief Complaint	"I have a bad headache and nausea."
Airway and Breathing	Airway is patent, respirations are increased, and tidal volume is adequate.
Circulation	Pulse is rapid, strong, and regular; skin is cool and diaphoretic.

1. What initial management is indicated for this patient?

_____

_____

_____

_____

The patient tells you that she woke earlier that morning, turned on the gas furnace, and went back to sleep. She was later awakened by her symptoms. You suspect a potentially toxic exposure and perform a focused history and physical examination **(Table 7-2)**.

Table 7-2 Focused History and Physical Examination

Substance	Possible exposure to carbon monoxide
When Did You Become Exposed?	"I guess while I was asleep."
Over What Period of Time Were You Exposed?	"About 2 or 3 hours."
Interventions Prior to EMS Arrival	None
Estimated Weight	125 pounds (57 kg)
Oxygen Saturation	98% (on 100% oxygen)
Breath Sounds	Clear and equal bilaterally
Blood Glucose	105 mg/dL
Pupils	Equal and reactive to light

ECG leads are attached to the patient's chest, and a 6-second rhythm strip is obtained for interpretation **(Figure 7-1)**.

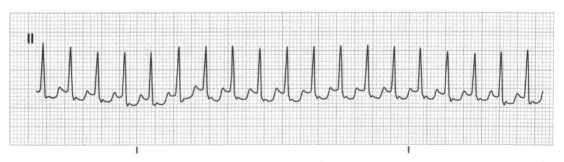

■ **Figure 7-1** Your patient's cardiac rhythm.

2. What is your interpretation of this cardiac rhythm?

_____

_____

_____

_____

An IV line of normal saline is initiated and set at a keep-vein-open rate. You obtain baseline vital signs and a SAMPLE history **(Table 7-3)** as your partner retrieves the stretcher from the ambulance.

Table 7-3 Baseline Vital Signs and SAMPLE History

Blood Pressure	130/86 mm Hg
Pulse	180 beats/min, strong and regular
Respirations	24 breaths/min with adequate tidal volume
Oxygen Saturation	96% (on 100% oxygen)
Signs and Symptoms	Disoriented, headache, nausea, tachypnea, tachycardia
Allergies	"I am not allergic to any medications."
Medications	"I take vitamins."
Pertinent Past History	"I do not have any medical problems."
Last Oral Intake	"I ate supper at about 8 pm last night."
Events Leading to Present Illness	"I turned on the gas furnace, went back to sleep, and was awakened a few hours later with a headache and nausea."

3. What is your field impression of this patient?

_____

_____

_____

_____

4. Are the patient's vital signs and SAMPLE history consistent with your field impression?

_____

_____

_____

_____

The patient agrees to be transported to the hospital. You place her on the stretcher, load her into the ambulance, and begin transport to a hospital that is approximately 10 minutes away.

5. What specific treatment is required for this patient's condition?

_____

_____

_____

_____

Supplemental oxygen at 100% is continued en route. After notifying the hospital of your impending arrival, you perform an ongoing assessment of the patient **(Table 7-4)**.

The patient's mental status has improved with the 100% oxygen; however, she still complains of a headache and slight nausea. Her vital signs remain stable, and her cardiac rhythm has improved **(Figure 7-2)**.

Table 7-4 Ongoing Assessment

Level of Consciousness	Conscious and alert to person, place, and time
Airway and Breathing	22 breaths/min with adequate tidal volume.
Oxygen Saturation	98% (on 100% oxygen)
Blood Pressure	134/84 mm Hg
Pulse	118 beats/min, strong and regular
Blood Glucose	107 mg/dL
Pupils	Equal and reactive to light

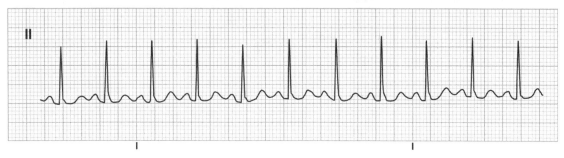

■ **Figure 7-2** Your patient's cardiac rhythm has improved.

6. Is further treatment required for this patient?

_____

_____

_____

_____

7. Are there any special considerations for this patient?

_____

_____

_____

_____

The patient is delivered to the emergency department. You give your verbal report to the attending physician, who immediately orders an arterial blood gas analysis.

The arterial blood gas analysis shows the following values: partial pressure of oxygen (PaO_2), 90 mm Hg; partial pressure of carbon dioxide (PCO_2), 42 mm Hg; oxygen saturation (SpO_2), 98%; and carboxyhemoglobin (HbCO), 34%. After further assessment and treatment in the emergency department, the patient is transferred to a nearby hyperbaric chamber.

Following treatment with hyperbaric oxygen, a repeat arterial blood gas analysis gives the following values: PaO_2, 100 mm Hg; PCO_2, 40 mm Hg; SpO_2, 98%; and HbCO, 0.02%. In addition, the patient's signs and symptoms have completely resolved. She is admitted to the hospital for observation and discharged the following day.

CASE STUDY ANSWERS AND SUMMARY

1. What initial management is indicated for this patient?

■ Give 100% supplemental oxygen via nonrebreathing mask
  • The patient's respirations, though increased, are producing adequate tidal volume; therefore, positive pressure ventilatory support is not required at this time.
  • Administer 100% supplemental oxygen as soon as possible to any patient with an altered mental status.

2. What is your interpretation of this cardiac rhythm?

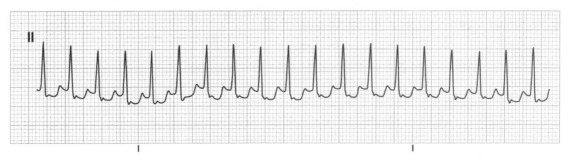

■ **Figure 7-3** Your patient's cardiac rhythm.

This narrow QRS complex tachycardia has a ventricular rate of approximately 180 beats/min **(Figure 7-3)**. P waves are not visible due to the rapid ventricular rate. This rhythm indicates a *supraventricular tachycardia.*

Supraventricular tachycardia (SVT) is an empiric term used to describe any narrow QRS complex rhythm with a ventricular rate that is 150 beats/min or greater. There are many variants of SVT, including atrial fibrillation with a rapid ventricular rate (RVR), atrial tachycardia, and junctional tachycardia. Because these rhythms typically have narrow QRS complexes, they are termed SVT, indicating that the primary pacemaker that initiated the cardiac rhythm is above (supra) the level of the ventricles. In this particular patient, SVT should be assumed to be the result of hypoxemia.

3. What is your field impression of this patient?

This patient is exhibiting signs and symptoms of *carbon monoxide toxicity.* The following assessment findings support this field impression:

■ Disorientation

■ Headache

■ Nausea

■ Symptoms began after turning on gas furnace

Carbon monoxide is produced by the incomplete combustion of fossil fuels, such as gas, oil, coal, and wood used in boilers, engine exhaust from automobile engines, solid fuel appliances (eg, gas furnaces), and open fires. Because this gas is colorless, odorless, and tasteless, it cannot be sensed by the patient and therefore is referred to as a "silent killer."

Though not physically harmful to the lung parenchyma itself, carbon monoxide dissociates (separates) oxygen from the hemoglobin (Hb) molecule, thus forming carboxyhemoglobin (HbCO). Once bound with carbon monoxide, hemoglobin is unable to transport oxygen, resulting in cellular and tissue hypoxia, metabolic acidosis, and organ dysfunction. Carbon monoxide will bind to hemoglobin 200 to 250 times more readily than oxygen.

The oxyhemoglobin (HbO_2) level, which is the percentage of oxygen bound to the hemoglobin molecule, does not contribute to the PaO_2. Only the physically dissolved oxygen in the blood plasma can create gas pressure and increase the PaO_2 level. This means that your patient can have a significantly low percentage of HbO_2 secondary to carbon monoxide toxicity and not manifest cyanosis.

Bright, cherry-red skin is an extremely late finding and generally is a precursor to death. Normal skin color, however, by no means rules out carbon monoxide toxicity.

The percentage of HbCO in an otherwise healthy person's blood can be gauged by signs and symptoms **(Table 7-5)**.

Table 7-5 Carboxyhemoglobin Levels Based on Signs and Symptoms

0%-10%	Typically asymptomatic
10%-20%	Headache, nausea, vomiting, loss of manual dexterity
20%-30%	Confusion, lethargy, cardiac dysrhythmias
30%-60%	Coma
Greater than 60%	Death

It is critical that you realize that the dissociation of oxygen and hemoglobin caused by increased levels of carbon monoxide in the blood is *reversible with prompt therapy.* Prolonged toxicity will result in irreversible cellular and tissue damage and eventual death. You must not delay definitive care of this patient!

4. Are the patient's vital signs and SAMPLE history consistent with your field impression?

The patient's blood pressure is unremarkable. However, her heart rate of 180 beats/min should be assumed to be secondary to hypoxemia and significant carbon monoxide toxicity. Tachypnea may or may not be seen in patients with carbon monoxide toxicity.

When the patient turned on the gas furnace, which probably had a leak in the line, carbon monoxide was emitted. This would explain her symptomatology. She is lucky that she woke up, as many patients quietly succumb to carbon monoxide poisoning in their sleep.

5. What specific treatment is required for this patient's condition?

- Give 100% supplemental oxygen via nonrebreathing mask
  - The most important treatment for this patient is 100% oxygen, which should be delivered until definitive care can be provided. To ensure maximal oxygen delivery, secure the nonrebreathing mask tightly to the patient's face.
  - Although currently the patient is breathing adequately, you must continue to monitor her for signs of inadequate breathing (eg, reduced tidal volume) and be prepared to initiate positive pressure ventilatory support.
- Hyperbaric Therapy
  - Hyperbaric therapy involves placing the patient in a pressurized chamber and delivering partial pressures of oxygen of more than 2,000 mm Hg (the equivalent of 3 atmospheres). The length of treatment ranges from 30 to 120 minutes, depending on the patient's HbCO level.
  - Hyperbaric therapy increases the amount of oxygen dissolved in the blood plasma and forces carbon monoxide from the hemoglobin molecule, thus allowing the blood to resume its oxygen-carrying capacity.

The longer HbCO is present and in significant quantity, the greater the tissue and cell damage. Therefore, the sooner you provide oxygen, the better! To emphasize the criticality of administering 100% oxygen and hyperbaric therapy, **Table 7-6** illustrates the half-life of carbon monoxide in the patient's blood, based on the patient's fractional inspired oxygen (FiO_2), or the percentage of oxygen that the patient is breathing.

Table 7-6 Half-life of Carbon Monoxide Based on the Patient's FiO_2

21% Oxygen	240-300 min
80% Oxygen	80-100 min
100% Oxygen	50-70 min
100% Oxygen at 3 Atmospheres (eg, Hyperbarics)	20-25 min

6. Is further treatment required for this patient?

Because the patient's clinical condition is improving (eg, improved mental status and ECG), only continual monitoring and oxygen therapy are required at this point.

7. Are there any special considerations for this patient?

When assessing any patient, especially one who has been potentially exposed to carbon monoxide, the paramedic must not rely solely upon the pulse oximeter as a true indicator of adequate oxygenation. It is, however, a useful tool in assessing the effectiveness of delivered oxygen therapy.

Pulse oximeters are blind to carbon monoxide. The dual wavelengths of infrared light they use to make measurements cannot distinguish between HbO_2 and HbCO, since the characteristics of the two are similar (eg, bright red). Furthermore, HbCO is combined with HbO_2 in the blood, which can produce a false reading suggestive of adequate oxygen saturation.

A patient could have blood concentrations of 15% HbCO (clinically significant) and 85% HbO_2 and the pulse oximeter would still indicate an oxygen saturation of 95%!

Remember, just like the cardiac monitor, the pulse oximeter is an electrical adjunct to a careful and systematic *physical* assessment of your patient. It is designed to show gross abnormalities, not subtle changes.

Another consideration in patients with carbon monoxide exposure is to ensure that all persons are removed from the environment in which the exposure took place. This may require notifying anyone at the patient's residence to evacuate the house.

Summary

Carbon monoxide toxicity should be suspected any time a patient complains of flu-like symptoms (eg, nausea, vomiting, or headache) following prolonged exposure in an enclosed space. Toxic environments can be created by obvious situations such as a structural fire, or less-obvious situations such as when a gas heating furnace has been turned on for the first time during the season. A classic finding of carbon monoxide exposure occurs when multiple patients in the same residence complain of the same or similar symptoms.

Carbon monoxide exposure results in cellular and tissue hypoxia because it binds to the hemoglobin molecule and forms HbCO, preventing the transport of oxygen throughout the body. The level of HbCO in the blood is measured with an arterial blood gas analysis.

The signs and symptoms of carbon monoxide toxicity depend on the level of HbCO in the person's blood and typically occur when the HbCO concentration is greater than 10%. Signs and symptoms range from headache, nausea, and vomiting to confusion, cardiac dysrhythmias, and coma. Cherry-red skin is an extremely rare, late sign of carbon monoxide poisoning and is a precursor to death.

Prior to initiating treatment, you must ensure your own safety and the safety of your partner by not entering the toxic environment without appropriate breathing apparatus or by limiting your exposure to the minimum possible.

The mainstay of treatment for carbon monoxide toxicity includes ensuring adequate oxygenation and ventilation and transporting the patient to a hyperbaric facility. There, pressurized oxygen is used to force the carbon monoxide from the hemoglobin molecule, thus allowing it to reunite with oxygen. If carbon monoxide toxicity is left untreated, the patient will die of prolonged cellular and tissue hypoxia.

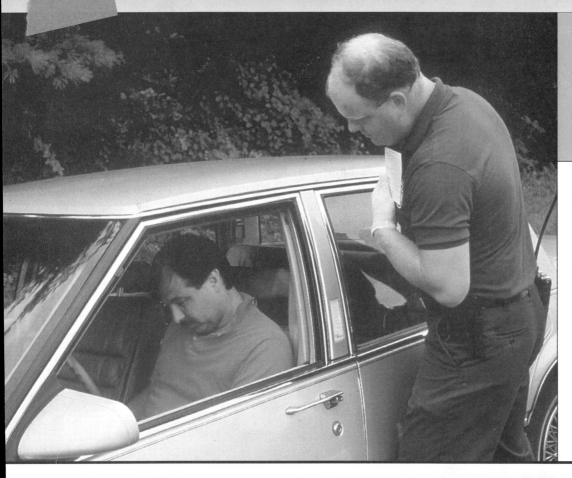

8

34-Year-Old Male Who Is Semiconscious

A concerned motorist called 9-1-1 because a man appeared to be unconscious in his car parked alongside the highway. You request that law enforcement respond to the scene prior to your arrival. The time of the call is 12:33 pm.

After securing the scene, a law enforcement officer advises you that the patient, a 34-year-old male, is semiconscious in his car. You and your partner quickly remove the patient from his car and perform an initial assessment **(Table 8-1)**.

Table 8-1 Initial Assessment

Level of Consciousness	Responsive to painful stimuli only
Chief Complaint	Altered mental status
Airway and Breathing	Airway is patent; respirations are slow and shallow
Circulation	Radial pulse is slow and weak; skin is pale and cool

1. What initial management is indicated for this patient?

_____

_____

_____

You perform a focused history and physical examination on the patient **(Table 8-2)**. Because there were no witnesses to this event, you are unable to obtain much of the needed information for your focused exam. The law enforcement officer tells you that he has found an empty medication bottle in the patient's car.

Table 8-2 Focused History and Physical Examination

Description of the Episode	Patient was found semiconscious in his car.
Onset	Unknown
Duration	Unknown
Associated Symptoms	Unknown
Evidence of Trauma	None
Interventions Prior to EMS Arrival	None
Seizures	Unknown
Fever	Patient is afebrile
Pupils	Bilaterally constricted
Blood Glucose	103 mg/dL

The fire department arrives at the scene to provide assistance. As one of the firefighters assists your partner in managing the patient's airway, you attach the cardiac monitor and obtain a cardiac rhythm tracing **(Figure 8-1)**.

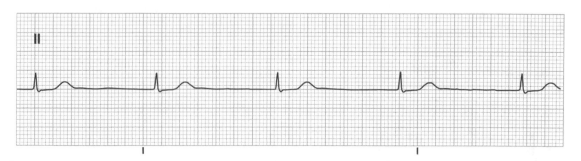

■ **Figure 8-1** Your patient's cardiac rhythm.

2. What is your interpretation of this cardiac rhythm?

_____

_____

_____

_____

The empty medication bottle found in the patient's car contains Dilaudid. It is prescribed to a woman and was filled 3 days earlier. The prescription is for 30 tablets.

As your partner and a firefighter continue to manage the patient's airway, you establish an IV line of normal saline. After securing the IV line, you obtain baseline vital signs and a SAMPLE history **(Table 8-3)**. The patient is unable to provide you with his medical history.

Table 8-3 Baseline Vital Signs and SAMPLE History

Blood Pressure	80/50 mm Hg
Pulse	46 beats/min, weak and regular
Respirations	Ventilated at 15 breaths/min
Oxygen Saturation	96% (ventilated with 100% oxygen)
Signs and Symptoms	Respiratory depression, hypotension, and bradycardia
Allergies	Unknown
Medications	Unknown
Pertinent Past History	Unknown
Last Oral Intake	Unknown
Events Leading to Present Illness	Unknown

3. What is your field impression of this patient?

_____

_____

_____

_____

4. Are the patient's vital signs and SAMPLE history consistent with your field impression?

_____

_____

_____

_____

The patient is placed on the stretcher and loaded into the ambulance. Your partner and the firefighter continue managing the patient's airway as you prepare for your next intervention.

5. What specific treatment is required for this patient's condition?

_____

_____

_____

_____

You see improvement in the patient's respiratory rate, vital signs, and cardiac rhythm **(Figure 8-2)** following your next intervention. The patient's level of consciousness has also improved, and he pushes the bag-valve-mask device away from his face. He will, however, tolerate a nonrebreathing mask with 100% supplemental oxygen.

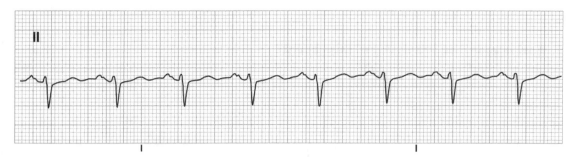

■ **Figure 8-2** Your patient's cardiac rhythm has improved.

You continue giving 100% supplemental oxygen as you proceed to the hospital. Although drowsy, the patient continues to talk to you and admits to trying to kill himself after losing his job the previous day. He also tells you that he took the Dilaudid from his mother.

You perform an ongoing assessment **(Table 8-4)** and then call your radio report in to the receiving hospital. Your estimated time of arrival is 7 minutes.

Table 8-4 Ongoing Assessment

Level of Consciousness	Conscious and alert, drowsy
Airway and Breathing	Respirations, 16 breaths/min; adequate tidal volume
Oxygen Saturation	98% (on 100% oxygen)
Blood Pressure	118/80 mm Hg
Pulse	78 beats/min, strong and regular
Pupils	Midpoint, equal and reactive
Blood Glucose	105 mg/dL

6. Is further treatment required for this patient?

7. Are there any special considerations for this patient?

The patient is delivered to the hospital in stable condition. You give your verbal report to the attending physician, who orders a toxicology screen of the patient's blood. The toxicology report reveals narcotics as well as traces of marijuana in the patient's blood. After further assessment and treatment in the emergency department, the patient is admitted to the hospital. The next day he is discharged to an in-patient drug rehabilitation facility.

CASE STUDY ANSWERS AND SUMMARY

1. What initial management is indicated for this patient?

- Positive pressure ventilation (bag-valve-mask device or pocket face-mask device)
  - Slow, shallow respirations (reduced tidal volume) are not adequate enough to support effective oxygenation of the blood.

- Airway adjunct
  - Because the patient is semiconscious and likely has an intact gag reflex, a nasopharyngeal airway should be inserted to assist in maintaining airway patency.

2. What is your interpretation of this cardiac rhythm?

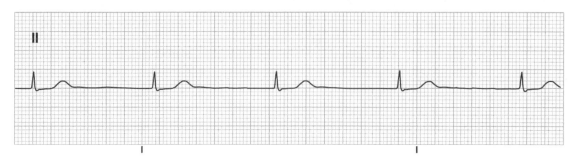

- **Figure 8-3** Your patient's cardiac rhythm.

This cardiac rhythm has a ventricular rate of approximately 45 beats/min **(Figure 8-3)**. The rhythm is regular, with narrow QRS complexes; however, there are no P waves preceding each QRS complex. This cardiac rhythm should be interpreted as a *junctional escape rhythm*.

Junctional escape rhythms occur when an ectopic pacemaker in the atrioventricular (AV) junction assumes control as the primary pacemaker for the heart at its inherent discharge, or escape, rate of 40 to 60 beats/min. These rhythms can occur when the sinoatrial (SA) node fails in its job as the primary pacemaker, or when the SA node's inherent discharge rate falls below that of the ectopic AV junctional pacemaker.

Junctional rhythms can occur with inverted P waves, without a P wave (buried in the QRS complex), or with P waves that follow the QRS complex.

Junctional rhythms are commonly caused by SA nodal disease, myocardial ischemia or infarction, and increased parasympathetic tone. In your patient, the rhythm is likely caused by CNS depression and hypoxia.

3. What is your field impression of this patient?

The patient's symptoms suggest *narcotic toxicity*. Hydromorphone (Dilaudid) is a powerful narcotic analgesic. The following assessment findings support a field impression of narcotic toxicity:

- Respiratory depression
- Bradycardia
- Hypotension
- Miosis (pupillary constriction)
- Depressed level of consciousness

Dilaudid is one of the most powerful prescription narcotics, making it a popular street drug. Because the Drug Enforcement Administration (DEA) tightly monitors both the prescribing and sale of Dilaudid, its street price is expensive relative to other narcotics, ranging from $40 to $60 *per tablet*. Dilaudid tablets, which are most often seen on the streets, are commonly referred to as "K-4s" because of the "K" on one side of the tablet, and the "4" on the other side.

Narcotic analgesic drugs depress the central nervous system (CNS), thereby relieving pain. When patients take these drugs in excessive amounts, undesirable effects such as respiratory depression, hypotension, and bradycardia are seen. If the patient is not treated promptly, death will occur, almost always as a result of respiratory arrest.

There are two classes of narcotics—opiates and opioids. Opiates contain or are extracted directly from opium. Opioids are synthetically produced, and have pharmacological properties similar to those of opium.

Narcotic analgesics include, among others, codeine (Methylmorphine), methadone (Dolophine), hydrocodone (Lortab), propoxyphene (Darvon), hydromorphone (Dilaudid), oxycodone (Percodan), meperidine (Demerol), and morphine (Morphine H.P.).

4. Are the patient's vital signs and SAMPLE history consistent with your field impression?

Hypotension, bradycardia, and respiratory depression are classic signs of CNS depression, which, in your patient, is caused by narcotic toxicity. You must remember that these clinical signs can be observed with an overdose of *any* CNS depressant drug, such as benzodiazepines and barbiturates, and are not exclusive to narcotics.

Because the patient is semiconscious, he is unable to provide you with SAMPLE history information. Although it is not possible in this particular case, you should attempt to obtain this information from family members, bystanders, or other people who are acquainted with the patient.

5. What specific treatment is required for this patient's condition?

■ Positive pressure ventilations (bag-valve-mask device or pocket-mask device)
  • Ventilatory support will ameliorate tissue hypoxia and help prevent respiratory and subsequent cardiac arrest. It is the most important initial treatment for patients with respiratory depression, regardless of the underlying cause.

■ Naloxone hydrochloride (Narcan) 0.4 to 2.0 mg
  • May be given intravenously, intramuscularly, subcutaneously, or intranasally
  • May repeat dose of 0.4 to 2 mg every 2 to 3 minutes. If there is no response after 10 mg, consider CNS depression from another cause.
  • Narcan is an opiate/narcotic antagonist that combines competitively with opiate receptors and blocks or reverses the actions of both opiate and opioid narcotic analgesics.
  • CNS depression may recur after the Narcan has worn off because the duration of action (half-life) of Narcan is shorter than that of narcotic analgesics.
  • Use Narcan with caution in patients who are known narcotic addicts, as CNS depression reversal may precipitate acute withdrawal seizures.

Naltrexone (Trexan) and nalmefine (Revex), although less commonly carried than Narcan, are also narcotic antagonists. You should refer to locally established protocols regarding the availability of these alternative drugs.

If the patient's condition does not improve after 10 mg of Narcan or an alternative narcotic antagonist, secure the airway with an endotracheal tube. Prolonged ventilatory support will be necessary until the cause of the CNS depression can be identified and definitively treated.

6. Is further treatment required for this patient?

No further treatment is necessary at this time. Continuously monitor the patient's level of consciousness, respirations, heart rate, and blood pressure in the event that he rebounds into CNS depression after the Narcan wears off.

7. Are there any special considerations for this patient?

The half-life of Narcan is shorter than that of narcotic drugs. Once the effects of Narcan wear off, CNS depression could recur, requiring additional dosing. Close patient monitoring for redevelopment of his original signs and symptoms is essential.

Ideally, Narcan should be titrated to improve the patient's ventilatory status, heart rate, and blood pressure. If possible, the patient should not be fully awakened in the field. Many times, narcotic reversal will wake up an extremely combative patient, who would pose a risk to your safety.

In patients who are addicted to narcotics, Narcan can precipitate acute withdrawal seizures and therefore should be used carefully. Signs of addiction include bruising along the course of a vein (needle tracks) and having previously treated the patient for a narcotic overdose.

Summary

Therapeutically, narcotic analgesics are effective in relieving acute and chronic pain. When these drugs are taken in excessive amounts, however, they can be deadly.

Narcotics depress the CNS and all the functions that it controls, including respirations, heart rate, and blood pressure. Death from a narcotic overdose is almost always the result of respiratory arrest.

Many narcotic analgesics are a combination of two drugs, one narcotic and one non-narcotic. For example, Lortab is a combination of hydrocodone and acetaminophen (Tylenol). An overdose of Lortab would result not only in CNS depression but potential acetaminophen toxicity as well. In an adult, a toxic dose of acetaminophen, 7 g, would result in liver failure.

Another combination analgesic, Percodan, is oxycodone and aspirin (acetylsalicylic acid or ASA). An overdose of Percodan would cause CNS depression and metabolic acidosis secondary to aspirin toxicity.

When responding to a call for a drug overdose, you must first ensure the safety of yourself and your partner. The situations in which drug overdoses occur often are violent or have the potential for violence.

Management of an overdose includes securing and maintaining a patent airway, ensuring adequate oxygenation and ventilation, and administering a reversal agent (such as Narcan). Consider intubation if a patient with CNS depression does not respond to a total of 10 mg of Narcan.

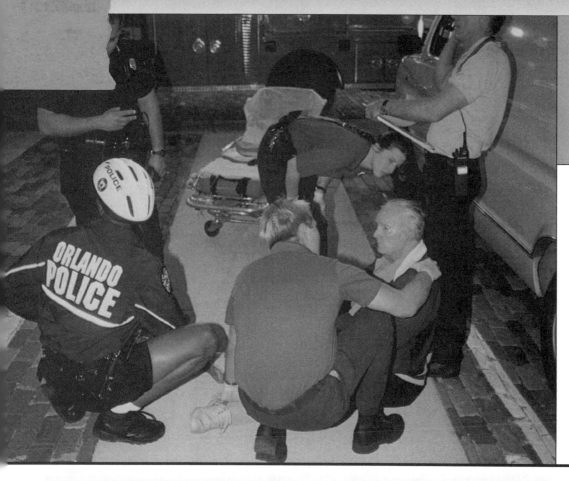

9

60-Year-Old Male with Confusion and Dehydration

At 10:45 pm, the police department requests your assistance at 3434 Main St, where they have pulled over a van for erratic driving. The driver, a 60-year-old male, told the police officer that he was on his way to the emergency room. Your response time to the scene is 6 minutes.

Upon arriving at the scene, you find the patient, who appears disoriented, sitting on the curb next to his van. He attempts to stand up, but gets very dizzy. As you begin your initial assessment **(Table 9-1)**, your partner obtains additional information from the police officer.

Table 9-1 Initial Assessment

Level of Consciousness	Disoriented
Chief Complaint	"I am weak, thirsty, and my stomach hurts."
Airway and Breathing	Airway is patent; respirations are increased with adequate tidal volume.
Circulation	Radial pulse is weak, irregular, and increased; skin is warm and dry with poor turgor.

1. What initial management is indicated for this patient?

_____

_____

_____

_____

Your partner performs the initial management for this patient. You obtain a focused history and physical examination **(Table 9-2)**, during which you note a strange odor on the patient's breath, but you are unsure if it is alcohol.

Table 9-2 Focused History and Physical Examination

Description of the Episode	According to the police officer, "The man was driving erratically. When I stopped him, I noticed that he was disoriented."
Onset	According to the patient, "This started 3 days ago and has gotten worse since then."
Duration	"I have been feeling bad for the last 3 days."
Associated Symptoms	"I have been urinating a lot, and am really dizzy."
Evidence of Trauma	None
Interventions Prior to EMS Arrival	None
Seizures	No seizures witnessed by the police officer
Fever	Oral temperature, 101.5° F
Blood Glucose	350 mg/dL
Pupils	Equal and reactive to light

Your partner attaches the ECG leads to the patient's chest, and obtains a 6-second strip of the patient's cardiac rhythm **(Figure 9-1)**.

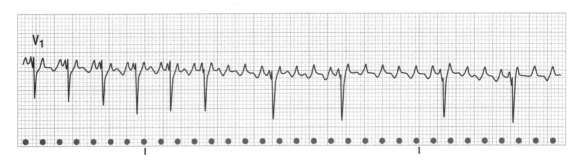

■ **Figure 9-1** Your patient's cardiac rhythm.

2. What is your interpretation of this cardiac rhythm?

_____

_____

_____

_____

The patient is moved into the ambulance to shield him from curious onlookers. Once inside, your partner initiates an intravenous line of normal saline with an 18-gauge catheter as you obtain baseline vital signs and a SAMPLE history **(Table 9-3)**. The patient hands you a wallet card containing his medical information.

Table 9-3 Baseline Vital Signs and SAMPLE History

Blood Pressure	88/56 mm Hg
Pulse	110 beats/min and irregular, weak at the radial site
Respirations	26 breaths/min, adequate tidal volume
Oxygen Saturation	98% (on 100% oxygen)
Signs and Symptoms	Disoriented, weakness, excessive thirst, dehydration
Allergies	Demerol and Motrin
Medications	Proscar
Pertinent Past History	"I had a heart infection a few years ago. I also have an enlarged prostate."
Last Oral Intake	"I don't remember when I last ate."
Events Leading to Present Illness	"I have been sick for the last 3 days. This all began when my stomach started hurting."

3. What is your field impression of this patient?

_____

_____

_____

_____

4. Are the patient's vital signs and SAMPLE history consistent with your field impression?

_____

_____

_____

You infuse 500 mL of normal saline to treat the patient's dehydration. Reassessment following this fluid bolus shows little improvement of his signs and symptoms, and he remains hypotensive and tachycardic.

5. What specific treatment is required for this patient's condition?

_____

_____

_____

You begin transport to the hospital, which is 8 miles away. Additional fluids are administered to the patient en route. You auscultate the patient's lungs, which are clear and equal bilaterally. You perform an ongoing assessment **(Table 9-4)** and then call your radio report to the receiving hospital.

Table 9-4 Ongoing Assessment

Level of Consciousness	Disoriented
Airway and Breathing	Respirations are 24 breaths/min, adequate tidal volume
Oxygen Saturation	98% (on 100% oxygen)
Blood Pressure	112/70 mm Hg
Pulse	88 beats/min, stronger, irregular
Blood Glucose	350 mg/dL
Fever	Oral temperature, 101.7° F
Pupils	Equal and reactive to light

6. Is further treatment required for this patient?

_____

_____

_____

_____

7. Are there any special considerations for this patient?

_____

_____

_____

_____

The patient's clinical condition and vital signs have improved upon arriving at the hospital. You give your verbal report to the attending physician, who orders a chemistry analysis of the patient's blood and an arterial blood gas analysis.

The patient is diagnosed with acute pancreatitis and new-onset insulin-dependent diabetes mellitus. He is given regular insulin followed by a continuous insulin infusion, sodium bicarbonate to treat the pH of 7.27, acetaminophen (Tylenol) for his fever, and additional IV fluids to correct his dehydration.

The patient is admitted to the medical intensive care unit, where the insulin treatment is continued, and his electrolyte imbalances are corrected. He is discharged home 2 weeks later with prescribed insulin and a follow-up appointment with an endocrinologist.

CASE STUDY ANSWERS AND SUMMARY

1. What initial management is indicated for this patient?

- 100% supplemental oxygen via nonrebreathing mask
  - Although this patient's respiratory rate is increased, his tidal volume is adequate. He does not require positive pressure ventilatory support at this time.
  - All patients with an altered mental status should be given 100% supplemental oxygen as soon as possible.

2. What is your interpretation of this cardiac rhythm?

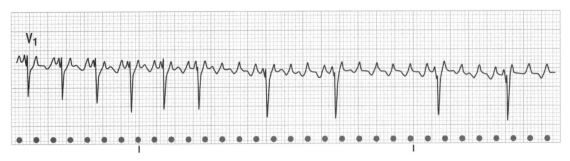

- **Figure 9-2** Your patient's cardiac rhythm.

This cardiac rhythm is irregular, with a ventricular rate of approximately 105 to 110 beats/min **(Figure 9-2)**. Instead of P waves, there are "F," or flutter waves, that make this rhythm consistent with atrial flutter. Since each QRS complex is not consistently preceded by the same number of flutter waves, making the ventricular rhythm irregular, this rhythm would be further interpreted as *atrial flutter with a variable block*.

Atrial flutter is caused by an ectopic atrial pacemaker outside of the sinoatrial (SA) node. The site of the ectopic pacemaker is commonly in the lower aspect of the atria, near the atrioventricular (AV) junction. The characteristic F waves, which take on a sawtooth appearance, make atrial flutter a relatively easy rhythm to interpret.

Chronic atrial flutter is most commonly seen in middle-aged and elderly patients. It is generally associated with conditions such as rheumatic heart disease, coronary artery disease, congestive heart failure, and damage to the SA node or atria from pericarditis or myocarditis. In some patients, atrial flutter may be idiopathic (of unknown cause).

Patients become symptomatic when atrial flutter is associated with a rapid ventricular rate (RVR). With rapid ventricular rates, especially those that are 150 beats/min or faster, the atria do not regularly contract and empty as they normally do during the end of ventricular diastole. This loss of "atrial kick" results in incomplete ventricular filling before they contract and may cause a reduction in cardiac output by as much as 25%.

In this particular patient, atrial flutter is most likely an indicator of a past medical problem, rather than a manifestation of his current condition.

3. What is your field impression of this patient?

This patient is exhibiting signs and symptoms of *diabetic ketoacidosis (DKA)*, which is also referred to as *diabetic coma*. Numerous assessment findings support this field impression:

- **Documented hyperglycemia** of 350 mg/dL. The normal blood glucose level ranges from 80 to 120 mg/dL.

- **Rapid breathing and acetone breath**, which are hallmark findings in patients with DKA. Sometimes mistaken for the smell of ethyl alcohol (ETOH), the odor on the patient's breath is caused by the removal of blood acetone via the lungs.

- **Frequent urination (polyuria),** which is secondary to a hyperglycemia-induced diuresis.
- **Generalized weakness,** which is caused by a lack of glucose (and energy) in the cells.
- **Signs of dehydration.** Increased blood glucose levels promote diuresis, which leads to dehydration. The patient has the following signs of dehydration:
  - Excessive thirst (polydipsia)
  - Poor skin turgor
  - Tachycardia
  - Orthostasis
    - Orthostasis is defined as a drop in systolic blood pressure of at least 15 mm Hg and/or an increase in the heart rate of 15 beats/min or more when the patient goes from a lying (or sitting) to a standing position. The orthostatic patient typically complains of dizziness upon standing.

DKA is a life-threatening complication of insulin-dependent diabetes mellitus (IDDM) and is characterized by hyperglycemia, severe dehydration, and metabolic acidosis.

IDDM occurs when the beta cells of the pancreas fail to produce adequate amounts of insulin, or cease to produce insulin altogether. Insulin is a hormone produced in the pancreatic beta cells that facilitates and regulates the uptake of glucose from the bloodstream and into the cell, where it is utilized in the production of energy. In the absence of insulin, the cells will starve for glucose **(Figure 9-3)**.

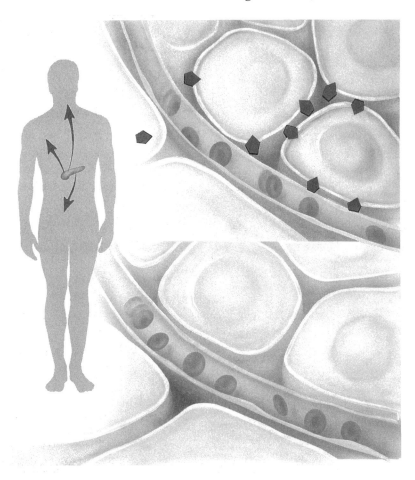

■ **Figure 9-3**
Insulin allows glucose to enter the cell.

Although the underlying etiology of IDDM is unclear, it may be associated with an infection (eg, pancreatitis), an autoimmune response in which antibodies destroy the beta cells, or a genetic predisposition that causes premature beta cell deterioration. The onset of IDDM typically occurs early in life; however, it can occur at any age.

Decreased insulin levels stimulate the release of large quantities of fatty acids from the fat cells into the blood. These free fatty acids are taken up by the liver where, in the setting of decreased insulin and increased glucagon, they set the stage for ketoacid production. Glucagon is a hormone that is produced in the alpha cells of the pancreas. This hormone stimulates the liver to produce glycogen, a complex sugar.

The elevated free fatty acids are converted to glucose in the liver through a process called gluconeogenesis. Unfortunately, since there is no insulin to facilitate cellular uptake, the glucose formed by gluconeogenesis remains in the bloodstream, which exacerbates the patient's hyperglycemia.

Elevated blood glucose levels prevent water reabsorption in the kidneys, which causes the body to excrete (diurese) large volumes of water. Excessive urination (polyuria) occurs, resulting in varying degrees of dehydration. Vomiting may also occur, which worsens the already dehydrated patient. Signs of dehydration include poor skin turgor, dry mucous membranes, and tachycardia.

Secondary to dehydration, the patient experiences an intense thirst (polydipsia). When massive amounts of water are excreted from the body, electrolytes such as sodium, potassium, and calcium are lost as well. Derangements in these critical electrolytes can cause life-threatening cardiac dysrhythmias, such as ventricular tachycardia (V-Tach) or ventricular fibrillation (V-Fib).

Polyphagia (intense hunger) and malaise (weakness) are also seen and are caused by cellular starvation from a lack of glucose.

When the cells do not receive glucose, the body switches to fat-based metabolism and produces ketones (ketoacidosis). As ketoacidosis develops and worsens, the respiratory system will attempt to compensate by increasing the rate and depth of breathing (Kussmaul's respiration), thus excreting excess carbon dioxide from the body and maintaining pH. The characteristic fruity odor on the patient's breath indicates the respiratory excretion of blood acetone, a type of ketone.

The signs and symptoms of DKA **(Table 9-5)** occur in patients with an established history of IDDM who have not taken their insulin or have inadvertently not taken enough insulin. They also occur as the initial presentation in a patient with new onset IDDM. In either case, they develop gradually and worsen over a period of 12 to 24 hours or longer.

Table 9-5 Signs and Symptoms of DKA/New Onset IDDM

The "Three Ps"
- Polyuria, polyphagia, and polydipsia

Signs of dehydration
- Warm, dry skin
- Dry mucous membranes
- Poor skin turgor
- Tachycardia
- Orthostasis

Altered mental status

Kussmaul's respirations
- Deep, rapid breathing with an acetone breath odor

Other signs and symptoms
- Abdominal pain
- Nausea and vomiting
- Malaise

4. Are the patient's vital signs and SAMPLE history consistent with your field impression?

The patient's low blood pressure and increased pulse rate are consistent with the dehydration associated with DKA. His increased respiratory rate, although not deep, indicates early Kussmaul's respiration, especially because of the acetone odor on his breath.

The events leading up to this patient's present illness (slow onset, abdominal pain) are consistent with pancreatitis. The heart infection that the patient referred to was most likely pericarditis or myocarditis. This history would explain his atrial flutter, as cardiac infections and subsequent SA nodal damage are common causes of this dysrhythmia.

5. What specific treatment is required for this patient's condition?

- **Ensure adequate oxygenation and ventilation.**
  - Administer 100% oxygen via nonrebreathing mask for the adequately breathing patient.
  - Provide positive pressure ventilatory support for the inadequately breathing patient.
- **Continually monitor the patient's mental status.**
  - Be prepared to intubate the patient to protect his airway if he becomes unconscious.
- **Give IV fluid boluses.**
  - Administer up to 2 L of normal saline to counteract the dehydration.
  - Reassess the patient and administer additional fluids if indicated.
- **Transport promptly for definitive care.**

Insulin is truly what this patient needs, but it is seldom administered in the field by the paramedic. If, however, transport to the hospital will be delayed, medical control may direct you to administer regular insulin to the patient. Sodium bicarbonate is also indicated if metabolic acidosis can be confirmed with an arterial blood gas analysis. Follow locally established protocols and contact medical control as needed regarding these pharmacologic interventions.

If a blood glucose reading cannot be obtained, and the patient is semiconscious or unconscious, draw blood for a red-top blood container and administer 25 g (50 mL) of 50% dextrose via IV push. This additional dextrose will not cause further harm, as it is negligible compared to what patients with ketoacidosis already have in their body. If the patient is hypoglycemic, however, dextrose may be life-saving. Remember the adage, when in doubt, give sugar!

6. Is further treatment required for this patient?

Because of the significant dehydration, this patient will likely require additional fluids while en route to the hospital. Additionally, continuous monitoring of his mental status is important. Perform another blood glucose check to ensure you report the most recent value to the emergency department physician.

7. Are there any special considerations for this patient?

As previously mentioned, electrolyte imbalances can and often do result from the massive diuresis associated with DKA. Specifically, derangements in serum sodium, potassium, and calcium can precipitate lethal cardiac dysrhythmias (V-Tach, V-Fib) and cardiac arrest. Continuous cardiac monitoring for warning signs of these dysrhythmias, such as premature ventricular complexes (PVCs), is important. Should cardiac arrest from V-Tach or V-Fib occur, defibrillation should be performed immediately.

Summary

DKA, also referred to as diabetic coma, should be suspected in any patient who is initially seen with hyperglycemia and signs of dehydration, such as tachycardia, poor skin turgor, and generalized malaise. The onset of DKA is slow, and gradually worsens over 12 to 24 hours, or longer.

DKA is a potentially life-threatening consequence of insulin-dependent diabetes mellitus (IDDM) and can occur if patients do not take their insulin or inadvertently do not take enough insulin. DKA can also be the initial presentation in a patient with new-onset IDDM. IDDM develops in most patients before age 19 years; however, it can occur at any age. Acute pancreatitis is a common precursor to IDDM.

In the absence of insulin, glucose pools in the blood and causes a variety of physiologic derangements. Blood glucose levels of 300 to 500 mg/dL are not uncommon in patients with DKA. Early signs of DKA include diuresis, which leads to dehydration. As DKA progresses, fat-based metabolism at the cellular level results in the production of ketones and the development of ketoacidosis. Furthermore, as a compensatory mechanism of the cell, gluconeogenesis occurs in the liver, which produces more glucose, thus worsening the hyperglycemia.

Later signs of DKA include severe dehydration, which may cause lethal cardiac dysrhythmias secondary to electrolyte abnormalities, alterations in mental status, and Kussmaul's respirations, a pattern of breathing characterized by deep, rapid respirations with an acetone odor on the breath. Kussmaul's respirations excrete excess carbon dioxide and blood acetone via the lungs.

Management of the patient with DKA begins by ensuring adequate oxygenation and ventilation. Fluid boluses, sometimes as much as 4 to 5 L, are required to counteract severe dehydration. If acidosis is documented, sodium bicarbonate will be needed to buffer the excess acid. Definitive care for the patient includes the administration of insulin, which is typically not performed in the field by the paramedic. If, however, transport time will be lengthy, medical control may direct you to administer regular insulin to the patient.

Failure to recognize and manage the signs and symptoms associated with DKA will result in the death of the patient due to profound metabolic acidosis and severe electrolyte abnormalities.

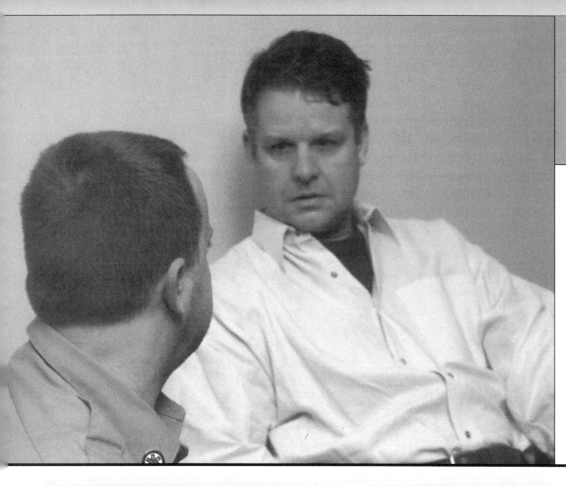

10

36-Year-Old Male Who Had a Seizure

At 4:44 pm, your unit is dispatched to 113 East Hosack for a 36-year-old male who is having a seizure. The call to 9-1-1 was made by the patient's frantic wife. Your response time to the scene is less than 2 minutes.

Upon arriving at the scene, you enter the patient's residence and find the patient sitting on the floor against a wall. You note that he is disoriented, agitated, and is incontinent of urine. The wife, who witnessed the seizure, denies any injury to the patient. After ruling out trauma, you perform an initial assessment **(Table 10-1)**.

Table 10-1 Initial Assessment

Level of Consciousness	Disoriented and agitated
Chief Complaint	According to his wife, "He had a seizure."
Airway and Breathing	Airway is patent; respirations are increased, adequate tidal volume.
Circulation	Radial pulse is weak and rapid, skin is cool and diaphoretic.

1. What initial management is indicated for this patient?

_____

_____

_____

_____

The appropriate initial management for this patient is complete. He remains disoriented and keeps asking you what happened. You perform a focused history and physical examination **(Table 10-2)**. The patient's wife provides you with the information you need.

Table 10-2 Focused History and Physical Examination

Description of the Episode	"He was reading the newspaper, when he suddenly let out a scream. I ran into the kitchen, and found him seizing in his chair. His entire body was twitching."
Onset	"This happened suddenly. He was fine up until this point."
Duration	"The seizure lasted for about 4 to 5 minutes."
Associated Symptoms	"None that I noticed."
Evidence of Trauma	None
Interventions Prior to EMS Arrival	"I moved him from the chair to the floor. I didn't know what else to do."
Fever	Temperature, 98.5° F
Blood Glucose	114 mg/dL

Following oxygen therapy, the patient's mental status has improved. He tells you that he has a seizure disorder from a closed head injury he sustained 8 years ago. The patient's wife hands you a bottle of the patient's phenobarbital. It was filled a week ago with 30 tablets and is still full. Your partner attaches the ECG leads to the patient's chest and obtains a cardiac rhythm tracing **(Figure 10-1)**.

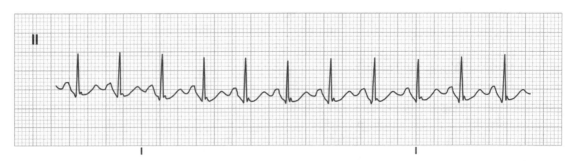

■ **Figure 10-1** Your patient's cardiac rhythm.

2. What is your interpretation of this cardiac rhythm?

The patient's mental status continues to improve. He is embarrassed about his incontinence, and asks his wife to get him another pair of pants. In the meantime, you obtain baseline vital signs and a SAMPLE history **(Table 10-3)**.

Table 10-3 Baseline Vital Signs and SAMPLE History

Blood Pressure	148/90 mm Hg
Pulse	128 beats/min, strong and regular
Respirations	22 breaths/min, adequate tidal volume
Oxygen Saturation	99% (on 100% oxygen)
Signs and Symptoms	Seizure
Allergies	"I am not allergic to any medications."
Medications	"I take phenobarbital for seizures."
Pertinent Past History	"I've had occasional seizures since that head injury."
Last Oral Intake	"I vaguely remember eating lunch about 2 or 3 hours ago."
Events Leading to Present Illness	"My wife tells me that I was reading the newspaper, when I suddenly screamed and had a seizure."

3. What is your field impression of this patient?

4. Are the patient's vital signs and SAMPLE history consistent with your field impression?

_____

_____

_____

The patient agrees to EMS transport to the hospital. After initiating an IV line with normal saline, the patient changes his mind, stating that he feels fine. You advise him that evaluation in the emergency department is necessary in order to determine what caused his seizure. As you are deliberating the issue with the patient, he complains of a "funny taste in his mouth" and immediately has another seizure.

5. What specific treatment is required for this patient's condition?

_____

_____

_____

Following administration of the appropriate pharmacological intervention, the patient's seizure stops. You continue to appropriately manage his airway as your partner retrieves the stretcher. The patient, who is still postictal, is loaded into the ambulance and transported to a hospital 15 to 20 miles away.

En route, you conduct an ongoing assessment **(Table 10-4)** and then call your radio report to the receiving hospital.

Table 10-4 Ongoing Assessment

Level of Consciousness	Postictal (confused, disoriented)
Airway and Breathing	Respirations, 24 breaths/min; adequate tidal volume
Oxygen Saturation	97% (on 100% oxygen)
Blood Pressure	148/88 mm Hg
Pulse	122 beats/min, strong and regular
Blood Glucose	124 mg/dL

6. Is further treatment required for this patient?

_____

_____

_____

_____

7. Are there any special considerations for this patient?

_____

_____

_____

_____

The patient is delivered to the emergency department. He remains postictal from the seizure; however, he is breathing adequately and his vital signs are stable.

You give your verbal report to the attending physician, who orders lab work to assess the level of phenobarbital in his blood. Subsequent results show his medication level to be subtherapeutic.

A computed tomographic (CT) scan of the patient's head is performed, which reveals no intracranial bleeding or space-occupying lesions. He is admitted for observation and regulation of his medications and is discharged home the next day without neurologic deficit.

CASE STUDY ANSWERS AND SUMMARY

1. What initial management is indicated for this patient?

- 100% supplemental oxygen via nonrebreathing mask
  - This patient is breathing adequately (adequate tidal volume); therefore, positive pressure ventilatory support is not required at this time.
  - During a grand mal seizure, the intercostal muscles and diaphragm are both paralyzed, which causes apnea and hypoxia. Providing 100% supplemental oxygen will ameliorate the hypoxia that occurred during the seizure.

2. What is your interpretation of this cardiac rhythm?

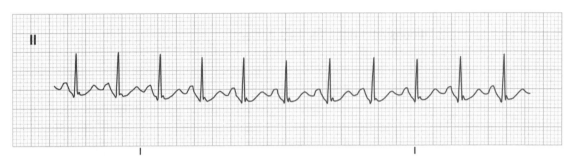

- **Figure 10-2** Your patient's cardiac rhythm.

This is a regular, narrow QRS complex rhythm, with a ventricular rate of approximately 125 beats/min **(Figure 10-2)**. There are monomorphic P waves that consistently precede each QRS complex. There are no premature complexes in conjunction with this rhythm, which indicates *sinus tachycardia*.

Tachycardia is a very common finding, both during and after a grand mal seizure. During the clonic phase of a seizure, which is characterized by an alternation of muscular rigidity and relaxation, there is a massive autonomic discharge of epinephrine from the sympathetic nervous system. This results in hyperventilation, hypersalivation, and tachycardia. Once the seizure ends, the epinephrine level in the blood decreases and the heart rate normalizes.

3. What is your field impression of this patient?

This patient has experienced a *grand mal seizure, secondary to noncompliance with his prescribed anticonvulsant medication.* The following assessment findings support this field impression:

- **Known seizure disorder** from a prior head injury
- **Full body "twitching"** is consistent with a grand mal (tonic-clonic) seizure.
- **Prescribed phenobarbital,** which was filled a week ago and is still full, suggests that this patient has not been taking his medication.
- **Urinary incontinence** is a common finding in patients during a grand mal seizure, and occurs during the tonic phase.
- **Agitation and disorientation** are typical of the postictal phase that follows a grand mal seizure.

A seizure is defined as transient alteration in a person's behavior or level of consciousness and is caused by a massive discharge of neurons in the brain. The exact pathophysiology of seizures is unclear, but they are believed to result from changes in the permeability of the neuron's membrane. Instability of the neuronic membrane alters the organized exchange of sodium and potassium, thus causing the neurons to depolarize chaotically.

There are many causes of seizures **(Table 10-5)**; however, ensuring adequate oxygenation and ventilation and terminating the seizure pharmacologically is more critical than trying to determine the seizure's exact origin.

Table 10-5 Common Cause of Seizures

Head trauma
Stroke (ischemic or hemorrhagic)
Hypoxia from any cause
Drug/alcohol overdose
Shock (hypoperfusion)
Metabolic derangements (hypoglycemia and hyperglycemia)
Space-occupying intracranial lesions (tumors)
Sepsis (massive infection)
Eclampsia

Generalized seizures include grand mal (tonic-clonic) seizures and petit mal (absence) seizures. The exact origin or focus of a generalized seizure is typically undefined; however, focal (localized) seizures may progress to a generalized seizure. Petit mal seizures typically occur in children between the ages of 4 and 12 years and are characterized by transient lapses in consciousness without generalized muscular involvement. A child who is "staring out into space" is a common description of a petit mal seizure. The seizure typically lasts less than 15 to 30 seconds and is followed by an immediate return to full consciousness. There is typically no postictal period following a petit mal seizure.

Grand mal seizures are common and are associated with significant mortality and morbidity. Oftentimes, grand mal seizures are preceded by an aura, which warns the patient of the impending seizure. Auras manifest differently and may include a strange taste (usually metallic) or an odd odor. Some people will complain of a strange feeling in their abdomen or, in the case of this patient, may suddenly scream.

The seizure itself begins with a sudden loss of consciousness, followed by the tonic phase, in which the muscles become tense and contracted. Tongue-biting and urinary or bowel incontinence may also occur during the tonic phase. The clonic phase of the seizure is characterized by rhythmic jerking movements of the extremities, and a massive autonomic discharge, which results in hyperventilation, hypersalivation, and tachycardia. A grand mal seizure is commonly referred to as a tonic-clonic seizure, because of the characteristic alternation in muscular rigidity (tonic phase) and flaccidity (clonic phase).

The intercostal muscles and diaphragm are paralyzed during a grand mal seizure, which causes hypoxia and cyanosis due to inadequate breathing or apnea. This is why death secondary to a seizure is most commonly the result of hypoxia.

Immediately following the seizure, the patient remains comatose and progresses into the postictal phase, characterized by confusion, agitation, combativeness, and, occasionally, transient neurologic deficits.

Status epilepticus is defined as a prolonged (≥ 30 minutes) grand mal seizure or two consecutive seizures without an intervening period of consciousness (lucid interval). Clearly, this is a dire medical emergency that requires immediate airway management and pharmacological intervention.

4. Are the patient's vital signs and SAMPLE history consistent with your field impression?

The elevated heart rate and blood pressure and increased respiration rate are consistent with the autonomic discharge during the clonic phase of the seizure. These values typically normalize after the seizure has ended.

We have already established a preexisting history of seizures. The events leading up to the seizure are consistent with an aura, and the patient's medication is a commonly prescribed anticonvulsant.

- **Phenobarbital** (Solfoton, Luminal) is a barbiturate that is commonly prescribed to patients with seizures.

Other medications commonly prescribed to patients with seizure disorders include valproic acid (Depakote), clonazepam (Klonopin), carbamazepine (Tegretol), and phenytoin (Dilantin).

5. What specific treatment is required for this patient's condition?

- **Protect the patient from injury.**
  - Move any furniture or other obstructions out of the way.
  - Protect the patient's head from striking the floor during the seizure.

- **Positive pressure ventilations (bag-valve-mask device or pocket-mask device)**
  - As previously mentioned, the patient is not breathing adequately, or is apneic during a grand mal seizure. Ventilatory support is required in order to maintain adequate oxygenation and minimize hypoxia.
  - Insert a nasopharyngeal airway to assist in maintaining patency of the airway.

- **Pharmacologic treatment of the seizure**
  - Common medications used to terminate seizures include:
    - **Lorazepam (Ativan):** 1 to 4 mg via slow IV administration over 2 to 10 minutes. This dose can be repeated in 15 to 20 minutes, to a maximum dose of 8 mg. If given intravenously, Ativan must be prediluted with an equal volume of normal saline.
    - **Diazepam (Valium):** 5 mg over 2 minutes via IV push. This dose may be repeated every 10 to 15 minutes as needed, to a maximum dose of 30 mg. Diazepam is incompatible with D_5W and must be administered into an IV line of normal saline.
    - **Phenytoin (Dilantin):** 1 g or 15 to 20 mg/kg via slow IV push. Do not exceed a total dose of 1 g or a rate of 50 mg/min. Repeat doses of 100 to 150 mg can be repeated in 30-minute intervals. Use an inline filter when administering Dilantin, and flush the IV line with 10 to 20 mL of normal saline, both before and after administering the drug.

Refer to your locally established protocols for treatment recommendations, as other medications may be used in the management of seizures. Remember, the longer a seizure persists, the greater the chance of hypoxic death!

Further management for seizures includes not restraining the patient in any way. The tetanic muscle spasms that occur during the seizure can result in long bone fractures if you attempt physical restraint. Additionally, you should never attempt to pry the patient's mouth open, as dislodged teeth and the associated bleeding can obstruct the airway or be aspirated into the lungs.

6. Is further treatment required for this patient?

Supplemental oxygen therapy should be continued postictally, and the patient should be placed on his side (the recovery position) to facilitate drainage of the oral secretions commonly produced during a seizure. Oropharyngeal suctioning may be needed to clear his airway of thicker secretions, as well as any blood if he bit his tongue during the seizure.

Cardiac monitoring should continue, and you should be alert for hypoxia-related cardiac dysrhythmias.

Closely monitor the patient's level of consciousness and have the appropriate pharmacological agent (Valium, Ativan, Dilantin) nearby should another seizure occur.

7. Are there any special considerations for this patient?

This patient has had two seizures within a very short period of time. Clearly, he is predisposed to another; therefore, close monitoring is essential.

You should avoid anything that could precipitate another seizure, such as the use of lights and siren and unnecessarily shining a light into the patient's eyes to check for pupillary response. Dimming the lights in the back of the ambulance should be considered as well.

Summary

Although there are many physiologic causes of seizures (structural and metabolic), the most common precursor is patient noncompliance with prescribed anticonvulsant medication.

Seizure-related deaths are the result of hypoxia, especially in those who experience status epilepticus, in which the prolonged seizure causes apnea and hypoxic brain injury.

Assessment of the patient who has experienced a seizure should begin by ruling out trauma that may have occurred during the seizure, determining whether a history of seizures exists, and ascertaining overall medication compliance.

If the seizure has stopped prior to your arrival, as typically happens, and the patient is postictal, ensure a patent airway and administer supplemental oxygen as needed.

If the patient is actively seizing, you must protect the patient from injury, ensure adequate oxygenation and ventilation, which may involve positive pressure ventilatory support, and terminate the seizure with an anticonvulsant medication such as Valium, Ativan, or Dilantin. Never physically restrain a seizing patient or place anything in the patient's mouth in an attempt to pry the teeth apart, as these actions may injure the patient.

Any patient who experiences a seizure, especially for the first time, should be transported to the emergency department for evaluation, which may include a CT scan of the head to rule out intracranial bleeding or a lesion. If the patient has a known seizure disorder, serum analysis of their prescribed anticonvulsant medication will also be needed.

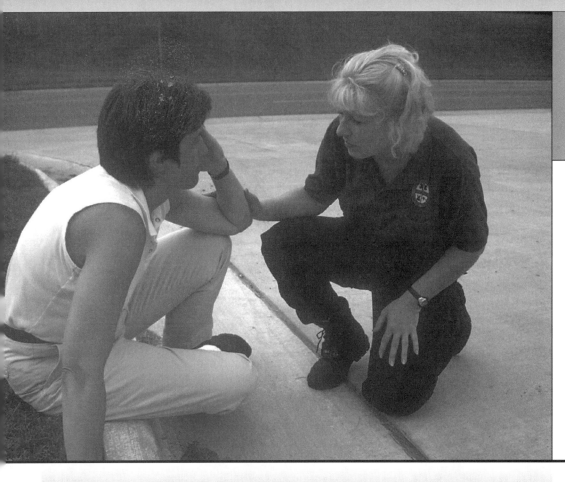

11

32-Year-Old Female with an Allergic Reaction

You are dispatched to 120 E Adler St for a 32-year-old female who is experiencing an allergic reaction. The time of call is 1:03 pm, and your response time to the scene is approximately 7 minutes.

You arrive at the scene at 1:10 pm, where you find the patient sitting alongside the driveway in front of her house. She is in obvious respiratory distress and is covered with a rash. As you perform an initial assessment **(Table 11-1)**, the patient tells you that she was stung by a hornet 15 minutes ago. Her respirations are labored; however, she has adequate tidal volume and is able to speak to you in full sentences.

Table 11-1 Initial Assessment

Level of Consciousness	Conscious, but restless
Chief Complaint	"I was stung by a hornet, and now I'm having trouble breathing. I have an Epi-Pen but it is expired."
Airway and Breathing	Airway is patent, audible wheezing is heard, and respirations are labored but with adequate tidal volume.
Circulation	Pulse is weak and rapid; skin is diaphoretic with a generalized rash.

1. What initial management is indicated for this patient?

_____

_____

_____

_____

After placing the patient on supplemental oxygen, an IV line of normal saline is established and set at a keep-vein-open rate. Following the appropriate pharmacological intervention, you conduct a focused history and physical examination **(Table 11-2)**.

Table 11-2 Focused History and Physical Examination

History of Allergies	"Yes, I am allergic to hornets, bees, and fire ants."
What Were You Exposed to	"A hornet."
How Were You Exposed	"It stung me."
Effects	"Shortly after I was stung, the rash developed. Then I felt tightness in my throat and could not breathe. Since you gave me that medication in the IV line, I can breathe easier."
Progression	"Within a few minutes of being stung, the rash developed, and then I began having trouble breathing."
Interventions Prior to EMS Arrival	"Nothing. I did not use my EpiPen because it was expired."
Breath Sounds	Scattered wheezing is heard on inhalation and exhalation.

Further assessment of the patient reveals mild facial swelling. Your partner attaches the ECG leads to the patient's chest and obtains a cardiac rhythm tracing **(Figure 11-1)**.

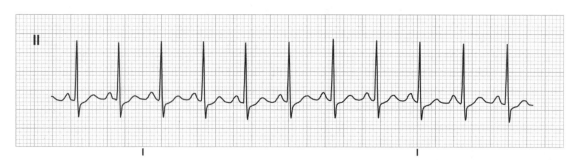

■ **Figure 11-1** Your patient's cardiac rhythm.

2. What is your interpretation of this cardiac rhythm?

_____

_____

_____

_____

As your partner retrieves the stretcher from the ambulance, you obtain baseline vital signs and a SAMPLE history **(Table 11-3)**. The patient is alert and oriented to person, place, and time, and is able to give you her medical information.

Table 11-3 Baseline Vital Signs and SAMPLE History

Blood Pressure	100/70 mm Hg
Pulse	132 beats/min, strong and regular
Respirations	22 breaths/min, slightly labored
Oxygen Saturation	95% (on 100% oxygen)
Signs and Symptoms	Respiratory distress, hives, facial swelling, all of which have improved since you administered the epinephrine.
Allergies	"I am not allergic to any medications. Just hornets, bees, and fire ants."
Medications	"I have a prescribed EpiPen but it is expired."
Pertinent Past History	"I do not have any other medical problems."
Last Oral Intake	"I ate lunch about 2 hours ago."
Events Leading to Present Illness	"I was stung by a hornet."

3. What is your field impression of this patient?

_____

_____

_____

_____

4. Are the patient's vital signs and SAMPLE history consistent with your field impression?

_____

_____

_____

_____

The patient's condition has improved significantly, but she still has a fine rash covering her body and complains of itching. You reach for the drug kit in preparation for your next intervention.

5. What specific treatment is required for this patient's condition?

_____

_____

_____

_____

You administer the next medication indicated for the patient's condition, after which you note that the rash is diminishing. You continue oxygen therapy and load the patient into the ambulance for transport to a hospital 7 miles away.

En route to the hospital, the patient's condition continues to improve. You perform an ongoing assessment **(Table 11-4)** and then call your radio report to the receiving facility.

Table 11-4 Ongoing Assessment

Level of Consciousness	Conscious and alert to person, place, and time, but appears drowsy.
Airway and Breathing	Respirations, 18 breaths/min; unlabored
Oxygen Saturation	98% (on 100% oxygen)
Blood Pressure	118/78 mm Hg
Pulse	104 beats/min, strong and regular
Breath Sounds	Bilaterally equal, scattered wheezing
Integumentary	Skin is somewhat flushed, rash has dissipated.

6. Is further treatment required for this patient?

_____

_____

_____

_____

7. Are there any special considerations for this patient?

_____

_____

_____

_____

The patient is delivered to the hospital in stable condition, and you give your verbal report to the charge nurse. The patient's signs and symptoms have completely resolved. Following additional assessment in the emergency department, she is given a nebulizer treatment and discharged home with a new prescription for an EpiPen.

CASE STUDY ANSWERS AND SUMMARY

1. What initial management is indicated for this patient?

- **100% supplemental oxygen via nonrebreathing mask**
  - Although this patient's respirations are labored and she has audible wheezing, she is conscious and alert, has adequate tidal volume, and is able to speak to you in complete sentences. She is not in need of ventilatory support at this time.
  - Closely monitor the patient for signs of inadequate breathing (shallow breathing, two-word dyspnea) and be prepared to initiate positive pressure ventilatory assistance.

- **An IV line of normal saline.**

- **Epinephrine, 0.3 to 0.5 mg (3 to 5 mL) of a 1:10,000 solution via IV push**
  - Epinephrine is the most important drug to give to patients with severe allergic reactions.
  - Epinephrine causes increased myocardial contractility (beta$_1$ effects), bronchodilation (beta$_2$ effects), and vasoconstriction (alpha effects), thus increasing blood pressure and improving oxygenation and ventilation.
  - IV epinephrine (1:10,000) is indicated for patients in shock, whereas subcutaneously administered epinephrine (1:1,000) is indicated for patients with mild to moderate allergic reactions, whose peripheral perfusion is adequate enough to effectively absorb the drug.

This patient is clearly in need of epinephrine to treat her condition or she will rapidly deteriorate. In many cases, life-saving treatment may have to be rendered prior to progressing beyond the initial assessment, especially if the patient presents with classic signs and symptoms of a life-threatening condition that you know requires a specific therapy. With this particular patient, you have gathered sufficient information from the initial assessment and general patient appearance to support the immediate administration of epinephrine.

2. What is your interpretation of this cardiac rhythm?

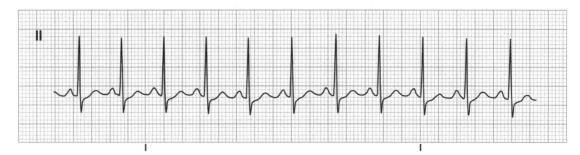

- **Figure 11-2** Your patient's cardiac rhythm.

This narrow QRS complex cardiac rhythm is regular, with a ventricular rate of approximately 130 beats/min **(Figure 11-2)**. There are upright, monomorphic P waves that consistently precede each QRS complex. This cardiac rhythm indicates *sinus tachycardia*.

With this particular patient, the tachycardia is caused by a sympathetic nervous system discharge of epinephrine as a compensatory mechanism to maintain perfusion. The epinephrine that you just administered to her is probably contributing to her tachycardia as well.

3. What is your field impression of this patient?

This patient is suffering from *anaphylactic shock (anaphylaxis)*, which is a life-threatening allergic reaction. Her condition has clearly improved following the administration of epinephrine. The following assessment findings support a field impression of anaphylaxis:

- **Known allergy to hornets**, exposure to which the patient has confirmed.

- **Generalized rash (urticaria)**, which is a hallmark finding in allergic reactions.

- **Rapid progression of symptoms** following the exposure, which is typical of a severe allergic reaction.

- **Labored breathing and wheezing**, which indicates respiratory compromise caused by bronchoconstriction and is also consistent with anaphylactic shock.

- **Tachycardia and restlessness**, which are signs of shock, and are typically not present during a mild or moderate allergic reaction.

Anaphylaxis, or anaphylactic shock, is the most serious allergic reaction and is caused by a massive release of antibodies in response to an antigen (allergen) that the immune system recognizes as being foreign.

People become allergic when they are "sensitized" to a specific antigen. When a foreign substance enters the body, whether by injection, ingestion, inhalation, or absorption, large amounts of IgE *(immunoglobulin E)* antibodies are produced by the immune system. Specific IgE antibodies are produced and released into the bloodstream for each antigen that the patient is exposed to. Therefore, a person with multiple allergies will have multiple IgE antibodies.

The IgE antibodies are released from the lymphatic system, where they bind to the cell membrane of circulating basophils and to the mast cells surrounding the blood vessels. There, they lay dormant until the body is exposed again to the same antigen.

If the patient is exposed to the same antigen a second time, the allergen cross-links at least two of the cell-bound IgE molecules though a process called "degranulation," causing the release of harmful substances such as histamines and leukotrienes (among others) from the mast cells and basophils.

Histamines cause multiple negative effects, one of which is the constriction of gastrointestinal and bronchiole smooth muscle, which increases gastric, lacrimal, and nasal secretions, resulting in tearing and rhinnorhea (runny nose). Histamines also promote vascular permeability and vasodilation. Increased vascular permeability allows plasma to leak into the interstitial space, which decreases intravascular volume and causes angioneurotic edema (subcutaneous swelling) that is commonly associated with airway closure. Severe vasodilation decreases right atrial preload and cardiac output, thus causing hypotension.

Leukotrienes cause profound bronchoconstriction and wheezing, which impairs oxygenation and ventilation, as well as coronary vasoconstriction, which may cause myocardial ischemia and cardiac dysrhythmias.

These chemical responses are responsible for the deleterious physiologic effects seen in patients with anaphylactic shock, the signs and symptoms of which are summarized by body system in **Table 11-5**.

Table 11-5 Signs and Symptoms of Anaphylactic Shock

Airway and Breathing
- Hoarseness or stridor
- Laryngeal edema
- Rhinnorhea (runny nose)
- Bronchospasm and wheezing
- Accessory muscle use and retractions

Cardiovascular
- Tachycardia and hypotension
- Chest tightness
- Cardiac dysrhythmias

Integumentary (Skin)
- Angioneurotic edema
- Urticaria (hives)
- Erythema and pruritus (red, itching, or burning skin)

Neurologic
- Headache
- Seizures
- Coma
- Anxiety and restlessness
- Dizziness, weakness, and syncope

Gastrointestinal
- Nausea and vomiting
- Abdominal pain
- Diarrhea

4. Are the patient's vital signs and SAMPLE history consistent with your field impression?

This patient's vital signs are consistent with shock, secondary to anaphylaxis. In addition, her oxygen saturation of 89% indicates that she is hypoxemic due to bronchoconstriction and impaired oxygenation and ventilation.

This patient has a clearly established history of allergies to hornets. Her prescribed EpiPen, although expired, confirms a previous exposure and allergic reaction.

5. What specific treatment is required for this patient's condition?

You have already administered epinephrine to the patient, which is clearly the most important initial drug. However, other medications are indicated for her condition, and are typically given in conjunction with epinephrine.

- **Diphenhydramine (Benadryl), 25 to 50 mg via IV or IM administration**
  - Benadryl, which is a commonly used adjunct to epinephrine, is an antihistamine that binds to both H_1 and H_2 receptors, thus blocking the release of histamines. Benadryl also blocks further histamine release from the mast cells and basophils.

On the basis of locally established protocols, additional pharmacologic agents may be used in the management of anaphylaxis. Corticosteroids, such as methylprednisolone (Solu-Medrol), or dexamethasone (Decadron) may be used to reduce the inflammatory response associated with anaphylaxis. Additionally, selective beta$_2$ agonists, such as albuterol (Proventil, Ventolin), or metaproterenol (Alupent) may be useful in relieving bronchospasm.

If the patient is severely hypotensive, vasopressor drugs such as dopamine (Intropin) or norepinephrine (Levophed) can be used concomitantly with epinephrine 1:10,000 and crystalloid (normal saline, lactated Ringer's solution) fluid boluses.

6. Is further treatment required for this patient?

At this point, the patient requires continuous monitoring to ensure complete resolution of her signs and symptoms. Medical control may order a nebulized bronchodilator (albuterol, Alupent) for continued scattered wheezing. A feeling of sleepiness or drowsiness is a common side effect following administration of Benadryl.

7. Are there any special considerations for this patient?

Although this patient does not have a cardiac history, you should monitor her blood pressure and heart rate, both of which have been increased by the epinephrine that you gave her. Catecholamines (epinephrine, norepinephrine) cause an increase in oxygen demand, which could exacerbate any underlying medical problems that the patient may have and be unaware of.

Summary

Anaphylactic shock is a life-threatening allergic reaction that can lead to death within a matter of minutes if not treated aggressively and immediately.

A person is predisposed to anaphylaxis after being sensitized to an offending antigen, such as insect venom (from a hornet, bee, or fire ant), medications (penicillin), or foods (shellfish). The sensitization process typically results in a limited allergic reaction, including urticaria, pruritis, and rhinnorhea.

Upon subsequent exposure, however, the signs and symptoms will be more severe, because the body has already developed IgE antibodies to the offending antigen and will release mass amounts of them in order to fight off the offending antigen. This mass release of IgE antibodies causes cardiovascular and respiratory compromise.

Signs and symptoms of anaphylaxis include urticaria, difficulty breathing, wheezing, facial and upper airway swelling, hypotension, and tachycardia.

The signs and symptoms of anaphylactic shock typically appear within a matter of minutes following exposure. Delayed reactions of up to 1 hour, however, have been observed.

In order to prevent cardiopulmonary collapse, treatment must be aggressive and immediate and includes ensuring adequate oxygenation and ventilation, positive pressure ventilation if breathing is inadequate, and early intubation if airway swelling is present. Pharmacological agents include epinephrine 1:10,000, Benadryl, and inhaled bronchodilators if needed.

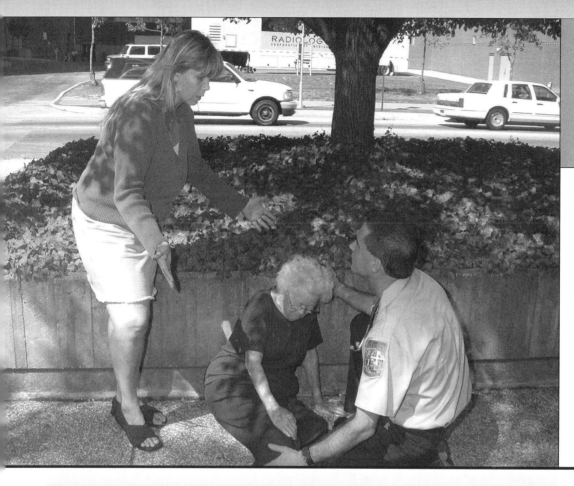

12

68-Year-Old Female with Palpitations and Dyspnea

The time is 10:45 am. The daughter of a 68-year-old female called EMS after her mother experienced a sudden onset of palpitations and dyspnea. The address is 1126 John's Rd, which is approximately 3 to 5 minutes from your station.

You arrive at the scene at 10:49 am, where you find the patient, who is in moderate distress, sitting on the sidewalk in front of her house. The patient tells you that she and her daughter were taking their daily walk when the symptoms began. After helping her mother sit down in the shade, the daughter called 9-1-1. You perform an initial assessment of the patient **(Table 12-1)** as your partner opens the jump kit.

Table 12-1 Initial Assessment

Level of Consciousness	Conscious and alert to person, place, and time
Chief Complaint	"My heart is fluttering, and I can't seem to catch my breath."
Airway and Breathing	Airway patent, respirations increased, tidal volume adequate
Circulation	Radial pulse weak and rapid, skin cool and diaphoretic

1. What initial management is indicated for this patient?

_____

_____

_____

_____

The appropriate initial management has been provided for the patient, who remains conscious and alert to person, place, and time. As you perform a focused history and physical examination **(Table 12-2)**, your partner attaches the ECG leads to the patient's chest.

Table 12-2 Focused History and Physical Examination

Onset	"This happened suddenly."
Provocation/Palliation	"My breathing gets worse when I try to walk, so my daughter helped me sit down."
Quality	"It feels like my heart is fluttering."
Radiation/Referred Pain	"I do not hurt anywhere."
Time	"This started about 15 minutes ago."
Interventions Prior to EMS Arrival	"My daughter helped me sit down. I was too out of breath to walk up the steps to my house."
Chest Exam	Chest wall moves symmetrically
Breath Sounds	Clear and equal bilaterally
Oxygen Saturation	97% (on 100% oxygen)

After completing your focused examination, your partner urgently turns your attention to the cardiac monitor **(Figure 12-1)**.

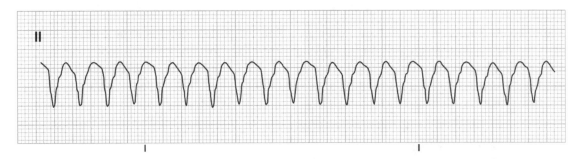

■ **Figure 12-1** Your patient's cardiac rhythm.

2. What is your interpretation of this cardiac rhythm?

_____

_____

_____

_____

After noting the patient's cardiac rhythm, you immediately reassess her. She remains diaphoretic and is now complaining of chest pressure. Her respirations remain adequate. Your partner establishes an IV line of normal saline as you quickly obtain baseline vital signs and a SAMPLE history **(Table 12-3)**.

Table 12-3 Baseline Vital Signs and SAMPLE History

Blood Pressure	80/50 mm Hg
Pulse	Rate too fast to count, quality weak
Respirations	24 breaths/min, adequate tidal volume
Oxygen Saturation	97% (on 100% oxygen)
Signs and Symptoms	Palpitations, hypotension, chest pressure
Allergies	"I am allergic to cefaclor and Demerol."
Medications	"I take torsemide and clonidine for my blood pressure."
Pertinent Past History	"I have high blood pressure and cataracts."
Last Oral Intake	"I ate a piece of toast 2 hours ago."
Events Leading to Present Illness	"I was walking with my daughter when this began."

3. What is your field impression of this patient?

_____

_____

_____

_____

4. Are the patient's vital signs and SAMPLE history consistent with your field impression?

_____

_____

_____

You explain to the patient the procedure that you are about to perform and why it is necessary. Your partner quickly retrieves the stretcher from the ambulance. The patient's daughter, who is upset at the situation, begins to cry. A neighbor, who became concerned and came over when she saw the ambulance, provides comfort and reassurance to the daughter.

5. What specific treatment is required for this patient's condition?

_____

_____

_____

Your initial intervention is unsuccessful in terminating this patient's cardiac dysrhythmia. After administering a pharmacologic agent, you repeat the procedure, and note a change in her cardiac rhythm **(Figure 12-2)**.

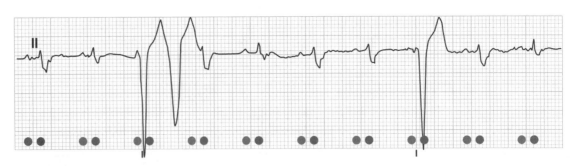

■ **Figure 12-2** Your patient's cardiac rhythm has changed.

With 100% oxygen therapy continuing, the patient, whose chest pressure and palpitations have resolved, is placed onto the stretcher and loaded into the ambulance. You initiate transport to the closest appropriate hospital, which is approximately 10 minutes away. En route, you conduct an ongoing assessment **(Table 12-4)** and then call your radio report in to the receiving hospital.

Table 12-4 Ongoing Assessment

Level of Consciousness	Conscious and alert to person, place, and time
Airway and Breathing	Respirations, 20 breaths/min; adequate tidal volume
Oxygen Saturation	98% (on 100% oxygen)
Blood Pressure	132/68 mm Hg
Pulse	98 beats/min, strong and irregular

6. Is further treatment required for this patient?

_____

_____

_____

_____

Further treatment is administered in order to prevent recurrence of her cardiac dysrhythmia. The patient is now displaying a normal sinus rhythm on the cardiac monitor. You note that her T waves are very small. Her vital signs and level of consciousness remain stable throughout transport.

7. Are there any special considerations for this patient?

_____

_____

_____

_____

You arrive at the hospital and give your verbal report to the attending physician. A 12-lead ECG is obtained, which reveals a normal sinus rhythm with flattened T waves and normal ST segments in all leads.

Blood chemistry results reveal a potassium level of 2.3 mEq/L (normal, 3.5 to 5.0 mEq/L). Following further assessment in the emergency department, the patient is diagnosed with hypokalemia, which likely resulted in her cardiac dysrhythmia.

She is administered the appropriate dose of potassium chloride and is admitted to the telemetry unit for observation. After adjusting the dose of her diuretic medication accordingly and prescribing a potassium supplement (K-Dur), she is discharged home 3 days later with a cardiology consult.

CASE STUDY ANSWERS AND SUMMARY

1. What initial management is indicated for this patient?

- 100% supplemental oxygen via nonrebreathing mask
  - This patient is not exhibiting signs of inadequate breathing (reduced tidal volume, altered mental status); therefore, positive pressure ventilatory support is not required at this time.
  - Administer 100% supplemental oxygen as soon as possible to any patient with potential cardiac compromise.

2. What is your interpretation of this cardiac rhythm?

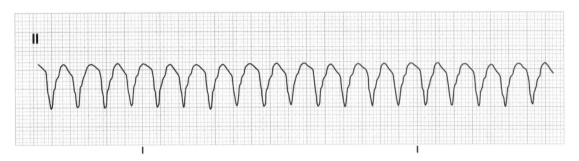

- **Figure 12-3** Your patient's cardiac rhythm.

This is a wide QRS complex cardiac rhythm **(Figure 12-3)**. It is essentially regular, with a ventricular rate of approximately 200 beats/min. The QRS complexes are consistently wide, bizarre, and monomorphic. There are no discernable P waves. This rhythm is consistent with *monomorphic ventricular tachycardia.*

V-Tach is a lethal cardiac dysrhythmia that originates in an ectopic pacemaker within the ventricles. This ventricular pacemaker site can be in the bundle branches, Purkinje network, or the ventricular myocardium itself.

As with any complex that originates within the ventricles, the QRS complexes of V-Tach are wide (> 0.12 seconds) and bizarre, with large T waves in the opposite direction as the main deflection of the QRS complex. The term monomorphic indicates that all of the complexes appear the same, both in width and direction.

V-Tach indicates significant myocardial irritability, and is commonly seen in patients with acute myocardial infarction, cardiomyopathy (progressive weakening of the myocardium), and left ventricular failure. A common precursor to V-Tach is prolongation of the QT interval, which can result from a variety of causes, including certain antiarrhythmic drugs (quinidine, procainamide), tricyclic antidepressant drugs (Elavil, Tofranil, Anafranil), severe bradycardias with accompanying AV heart block, and electrolyte disturbances (hypokalemia, hypomagnesemia).

V-Tach is frequently associated with hemodynamic instability (hypotension, chest pain, altered mental status) and can quickly deteriorate to ventricular fibrillation (V-Fib) and cardiac arrest unless promptly treated.

3. What is your field impression of this patient?

We have already established that the patient is in monomorphic V-Tach; however, due to her serious signs and symptoms linked to the tachycardia, she is *hemodynamically unstable* and will require immediate intervention. The following signs and symptoms indicate her hemodynamic instability:

- Dyspnea on exertion
- Chest pressure
- Hypotension

V-Tach frequently causes hemodynamic compromise. Since the ventricles are acting as the dominant pacemaker, atrial contraction and the subsequent volume of blood ejected into the ventricles are minimal. Additionally, there is not enough time for adequate ventricular filling because the ventricles are beating so quickly, so stroke volume decreases. These effects cause decreased cardiac output and hypotension.

The chest pressure that this patient is experiencing is caused by myocardial ischemia. This means that diminished cardiac output is not allowing adequate coronary blood flow to accommodate the patient's myocardial oxygen demand. When this happens, ischemic chest pain or pressure develops.

Dyspnea could be the result of anxiety from the palpitations or regurgitation of blood into the lungs secondary to impaired left ventricular function.

If cerebral perfusion diminishes, even slightly, the patient's mental status will become altered, ranging from confusion and disorientation to unconsciousness.

V-Tach has a high propensity for deteriorating to V-Fib and cardiac arrest; therefore, patients with V-Tach require treatment whether they are hemodynamically stable or not.

Although other conditions can cause a wide QRS complex tachycardia, such as supraventricular tachycardia with an intraventricular conduction delay (eg, bundle branch block), any wide complex tachycardia, especially in the presence of serious signs and symptoms, should be treated as V-Tach. In fact, 90% of wide complex tachycardias are indeed V-Tach.

4. Are the patient's vital signs and SAMPLE history consistent with your field impression?

The patient's hypotension and chest pressure are serious signs that indicate hemodynamic compromise. This is consistent with a field impression of unstable V-Tach.

The patient's history of hypertension could be a predisposing factor in causing V-Tach. Her medication allergies are probably not contributing to her present condition. Cefaclor (Ceclor) is a cephalosporin antibiotic, and meperidine (Demerol) is a narcotic analgesic.

She does, however, take torsemide (Demadex), which is a loop diuretic commonly prescribed in conjunction with antihypertensive medications (eg, clonidine). In addition to excreting water from the body, electrolytes such as sodium, potassium, and magnesium are lost as well in patients who take diuretic medications.

Electrolyte derangements (hyponatremia, hypokalemia, hypomagnesemia) can cause abnormalities in the cardiac electrical conduction system, with resultant cardiac dysrhythmias, such as PVCs, V-Tach, and V-Fib.

Perhaps this patient's electrolytes are abnormal secondary to taking diuretics and recent exercise, which also causes loss of water from the body.

5. What specific treatment is required for this patient's condition?

- **Synchronized cardioversion**
  - When cardioverting an unstable patient with V-Tach, start with 100 joules. If this is unsuccessful, repeat as needed at 200, 300, and 360 joules, respectively.
  - Assess the patient's cardiac rhythm and condition following each cardioversion. Be prepared to turn the synchronizer off and defibrillate immediately if V-Fib and cardiac arrest develop.
    - Unless the patient is unconscious, she should be sedated prior to cardioversion. Benzodiazepines, which induce a hypnotic-amnesiac effect, are commonly used for this purpose.
      - **Midazolam** (Versed) 1.0 to 2.5 mg via slow IV push.
      - **Diazepam** (Valium) 5 to 15 mg via slow IV push

The following antiarrhythmic medications may be used in conjunction with synchronized cardioversion, as well as to prevent the recurrence of V-Tach following successful cardioversion:

- **Amiodarone, 150 mg via fast IV infusion (over 10 minutes)**
  - Dilute the amiodarone in 20 to 30 mL of D_5W prior to administration.
    - Maintenance infusion during a 24-hour period is 360 mg over the first 6 hours (1.0 mg/min), then 540 mg over the remaining 18 hours (0.5 mg/min).
    - Maximum cumulative dose is 2.2 g in a 24-hour period.

- **Lidocaine, 1.0 to 1.5 mg/kg IV push**
  - Repeat every 5 to 10 minutes at 0.5 to 0.75 mg/kg
  - Maximum total dose of 3 mg/kg
  - Maintenance infusion is 1 to 4 mg/min.
    - Reduce the maintenance dose of lidocaine by 50% in patients older than 70 years and in patients with renal or hepatic dysfunction.

- **Procainamide, 20 mg/min via IV infusion**
  - Discontinue procainamide if the dysrhythmia is suppressed, hypotension develops, the QRS complex widens by more than 50% of its pretreatment width, or a total dose of 17 mg/kg has been given.
  - Maintenance infusion is 1 to 4 mg/min.

Follow locally established protocols regarding the use of antiarrhythmic medications in conjunction with, or following, successful cardioversion.

6. Is further treatment required for this patient?

The patient's hemodynamic status has improved significantly; however, her cardiac rhythm still suggests ventricular irritability (PVCs) and a strong possibility of recurrent V-Tach. If not already administered, an antiarrhythmic medication bolus (amiodarone, lidocaine, procainamide), followed by a maintenance infusion would be appropriate.

Ordinarily, PVCs are not treated pharmacologically, unless associated with hemodynamic compromise, or in the setting of acute myocardial infarction. However, in order to prevent a recurrence of V-Tach, it would be advisable in this patient. Contact medical control or refer to locally established protocols regarding the treatment of PVCs.

7. Are there any special considerations for this patient?

Until the underlying etiology that caused this patient's ventricular tachycardia can be identified and treated definitively, she is clearly at risk for redevelopment of V-Tach, which could deteriorate to V-Fib and cardiac arrest. You must be prepared to repeat cardioversion or defibrillate the patient if the need arises.

Continuous cardiac monitoring in this patient is critical in being able to identify warning signs of impending V-Tach or V-Fib, such as multiple PVCs (> 6 per min), polymorphic PVCs, or PVCs that fall on the downslope of the T wave (R on T phenomenon).

Summary

V-Tach is a lethal ventricular dysrhythmia, the underlying cause of which can be multifactorial, including cardiac ischemia or infarction, cardiomyopathy, and electrolyte abnormalities. In some patients, V-Tach may be idiopathic (of unknown cause). Without prompt treatment, deterioration to V-Fib and cardiac arrest could occur. The rhythm itself is characterized by wide (> 0.12 sec), bizarre QRS complexes, T waves in the opposite direction of the main QRS vector, and a ventricular rate that can range from 100 to 300 beats/min.

Assessment of the patient with V-Tach begins by determining if serious signs and symptoms exist, such as chest pain or pressure, shortness of breath, or hypotension. If the patient is hemodynamically stable, antiarrhythmic agents are generally used in the initial management. However, if the ventricular rate is greater than 150 beats/min, even without serious signs and symptoms, sedation followed by synchronized cardioversion may be used as the initial intervention.

If serious signs and symptoms linked to the tachycardia are present, synchronized cardioversion is indicated as the initial treatment. Unless the patient is unconscious, sedation with a benzodiazepine should be administered prior to the cardioversion.

Antiarrhythmic drugs may be used in conjunction with cardioversion, and as an adjunct to prevent recurrent V-Tach following successful termination of the dysrhythmia with cardioversion.

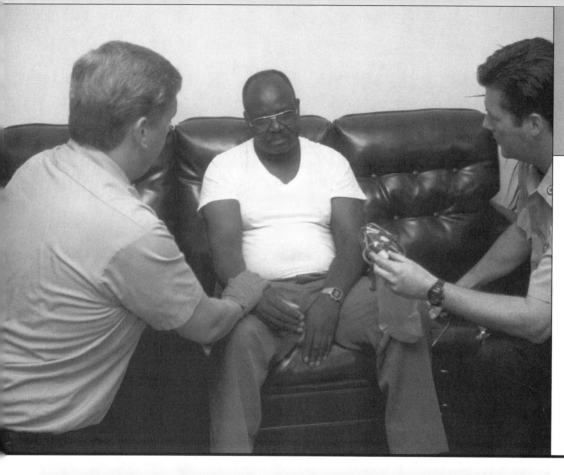

CASE STUDY

13

57-Year-Old Male with Weakness and Dyspnea

At 7:45 pm, you are dispatched to a residence at 214 Roadrunner Ln, for a 57-year-old male who is complaining of weakness and dyspnea. Your response time to the scene is approximately 8 minutes.

You arrive at the scene at 7:53 pm. You are met at the door by a woman, the patient's wife, who escorts you to her husband. You find the patient sitting on the couch in the living room. He is conscious, diaphoretic, and in moderate respiratory distress. You introduce yourself to the patient and perform an initial assessment (Table 13-1).

Table 13-1 Initial Assessment

Level of Consciousness	Conscious and alert to person, place, and time
Chief Complaint	"I am really weak and cannot catch my breath."
Airway and Breathing	Airway, patent; slightly increased and mildly labored respirations
Circulation	Radial pulse, slow and weak; skin, cool and diaphoretic

1. What initial management is indicated for this patient?

_____

_____

_____

_____

Your partner performs the appropriate initial management. The patient remains conscious and alert to person, place, and time and provides the information needed for the focused history and physical examination **(Table 13-2)**.

Table 13-2 Focused History and Physical Examination

Onset	"This began quite suddenly and has progressively worsened."
Provocation/Palliation	"Nothing that I do makes this any better or worse."
Quality	"I feel like I am smothering."
Radiation/Referred Pain	"I am not having any pain."
Time	"This started about 6 hours ago."
Interventions Prior to EMS Arrival	None
Chest Exam	Chest wall moves symmetrically, mild intercostal retractions noted
Breath Sounds	Scattered rales throughout all lung fields
Oxygen Saturation	97% (on 100% oxygen)
Blood Glucose	98 mg/dL
Pupils	Equal and reactive to light

Your patient attaches the ECG leads to the patient's chest and obtains a 6-second cardiac rhythm tracing **(Figure 13-1)**. The patient mentions to you that he has high blood pressure.

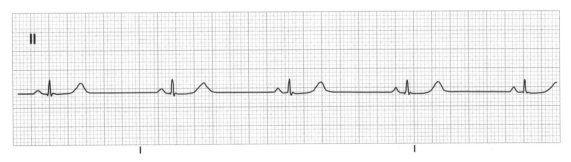

■ **Figure 13-1** Your patient's cardiac rhythm.

2. What is your interpretation of this cardiac rhythm?

You obtain baseline vital signs and a SAMPLE history **(Table 13-3)** as your partner is opening up the IV starter kit. The patient tells you that he is becoming nauseated.

Table 13-3 Baseline Vital Signs and SAMPLE History

Blood Pressure	88/60 mm Hg
Pulse	44 beats/min, weak and regular
Respirations	24 breaths/min and mildly labored
Oxygen Saturation	97% (on 100% oxygen)
Signs and Symptoms	Weakness, dyspnea, nausea
Allergies	"I am allergic to codeine and penicillin."
Medications	"I take Lopressor and Maxzide for my blood pressure."
Pertinent Past History	"I have high blood pressure."
Last Oral Intake	"I ate breakfast this morning. I was not hungry at supper, because I was not feeling well."
Events Leading to Present Illness	"The only thing that I can recall before this started was taking my blood pressure medicine."

3. What is your field impression of this patient?

4. Are the patient's vital signs and SAMPLE history consistent with your field impression?

_____

_____

_____

_____

An IV line of normal saline has been successfully established and is set at a keep-vein-open rate. You explain the procedure that you are about to perform to the patient, who is still conscious and alert to person, place, and time.

5. What specific treatment is required for this patient's condition?

_____

_____

_____

_____

Following the maximum dose of your initial pharmacologic intervention, the patient's condition remains unchanged. You quickly place the pacing pads on the patient's chest, load him into the ambulance, and transport to a hospital 15 miles away. While attempting cardiac pacing en route, you perform an ongoing assessment (Table 13-4).

Table 13-4 Ongoing Assessment

Level of Consciousness	Conscious and alert to person, place, and time
Airway and Breathing	Respirations, 24 breaths/min and mildly labored
Oxygen Saturation	96% (on 100% oxygen)
Blood Pressure	84/58 mm Hg
Pulse	46 beats/min, weak and regular
Blood Glucose	100 mg/dL
Pupils	Equal and reactive to light

Cardiac pacing is not successful for this patient. As you are picking up the cellular phone to call medical control, the patient tells you that he missed the last 4 doses of his Lopressor, so in an attempt to "catch himself up," he quadrupled his usual daily dose today. After staring at the patient in disbelief for a few seconds, you gently hang up the phone.

6. Is further treatment required for this patient?

_____

_____

_____

_____

After administering the drug that is most appropriate for this patient's condition, you note marked improvement within 5 minutes! The patient tells you that his breathing is "much easier," and that he is no longer nauseated. His vital signs and cardiac rhythm **(Figure 13-2)** have both improved as well.

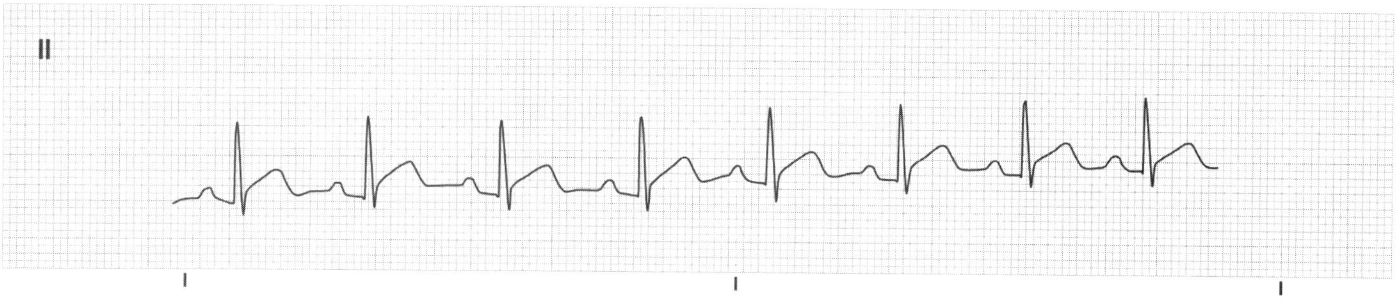

■ **Figure 13-2** Your patient's cardiac rhythm has improved.

After explaining to the patient what he has inadvertently done, he embarrassingly looks up at you and says, "Oops." You call your radio report to the receiving facility, with an estimated time of arrival of approximately 3 minutes.

7. Are there any special considerations for this patient?

_____

_____

_____

_____

The patient's condition continues to improve throughout transport, and he is delivered to the emergency department in stable condition. You give your verbal report to the attending physician. The patient is admitted overnight for observation and is discharged home the following day, with _explicitly clear instructions on the proper use of his prescribed medications._

CASE STUDY ANSWERS AND SUMMARY

1. What initial management is indicated for this patient?

- 100% supplemental oxygen via nonrebreathing mask
  - Although the patient's breathing is slightly increased and labored, he is conscious and alert and talking to you without difficulty. Positive pressure ventilatory support is not required at this time.
  - Any patient who complains of breathing difficulty should receive 100% supplemental oxygen as soon as possible.

2. What is your interpretation of this cardiac rhythm?

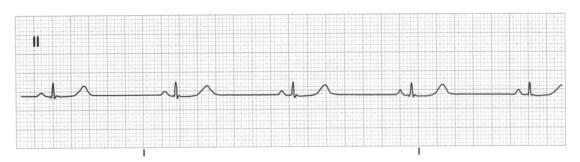

- **Figure 13-3** Your patient's cardiac rhythm.

This cardiac rhythm is regular and slow, with a ventricular rate of approximately 45 beats/min **(Figure 13-3)**. P waves are present, monomorphic, and are consistently followed by a narrow QRS complex. All of the characteristic components of a *sinus bradycardia* are present with this rhythm.

Sinus bradycardia is caused by increased parasympathetic nervous system stimulation and a resultant increase in the production of acetylcholine, the chemical mediator that regulates the parasympathetic nervous system. Acetylcholine acts upon the vagus nerve, which decreases the sinoatrial (SA) node discharge rate, slows conduction through the atrioventricular (AV) node, and decreases the heart rate.

Sinus bradycardia can either be absolute, in which the heart rate is less than 60 beats/min, or relative, in which the patient's heart rate is slower than would be expected for the condition.

There are many potential underlying causes of sinus bradycardia, including acute myocardial infarction (especially of the inferior wall), medication effects (digitalis, beta blockers), and diseases of the SA node. In some patients, especially those who are well-conditioned, sinus bradycardia may be a normal finding.

3. What is your field impression of this patient?

This patient is suffering from *symptomatic bradycardia*. The following signs and symptoms, which are linked to the bradycardia, support this field impression:

- Hypotension
- Dyspnea

When a patient is initially seen with a bradycardic rhythm, you must perform a systematic assessment in order to identify serious signs and symptoms that are linked to the bradycardia, as treatment will differ significantly from that of the stable patient.

Serious signs and symptoms include chest pain or pressure, shortness of breath, hypotension, altered mental status, and pulmonary edema.

When the heart beats too slowly, cardiac output, which is the volume of blood that is ejected from the left ventricle each minute, falls. Even if the patient's stroke volume (milliliters of blood ejected from the ventricles per beat), is adequate, the slow-beating heart is not pumping enough blood to the body per minute. Remember that cardiac output can fall as the result of decreased stroke volume, heart rate, or both.

Cardiac output = Stroke volume × Heart rate

This decrease in cardiac output can cause a variety of problems for the patient, including hypotension, which indicates systemic hypoperfusion, shortness of breath with pulmonary edema, indicating that blood is backing up into the lungs, and an altered mental status caused by cerebral hypoperfusion.

4. Are the patient's vital signs and SAMPLE history consistent with your field impression?

The patient's vital signs, specifically the low blood pressure and labored respirations, indicate hemodynamic instability and are thus consistent with your field impression of symptomatic bradycardia.

The patient has a history of hypertension, for which he takes metoprolol (Lopressor), a beta-adrenergic antagonist (beta-blocker). Even in therapeutic doses, some beta-blocking drugs can result in an undesirable bradycardia, with resultant hypotension. Perhaps there is a link between the beta-blocker medication and the patient's present condition.

5. What specific treatment is required for this patient's condition?

- **Atropine sulfate, 0.5 to 1.0 mg via rapid IV push**
  - Atropine is a parasympatholytic (vagolytic) drug that blocks the effects of acetylcholine on the vagus nerve within the parasympathetic nervous system (PNS). Acetylcholine is the chief chemical neurotransmitter of the PNS, which is why the PNS is commonly referred to as the cholinergic nervous system. The vagolytic effects of atropine increase the discharge rate of the SA node and enhance conduction through the AV junction.
  - Atropine exerts its effects on the supraventricular myocardium. It does not act upon the ventricles directly. If the AV junction is not blocked, the increase in SA nodal discharge will traverse the AV junction as usual and increase the ventricular rate. For this reason, atropine is generally not effective in treating bradycardias associated with an AV heart block, specifically, second-degree type II and third-degree AV block.
  - In patients with a pulse, 0.5 mg of atropine is generally given, followed by a reassessment. If the patient remains symptomatic, administration of atropine can be repeated at 3-minute to 5-minute intervals, until the maximum vagolytic dose of 0.04 mg/kg has been administered.
  - Atropine is also given to patients in asystole and to those who are initially seen with bradycardic (< 60 beats/min) pulseless electrical activity (PEA). These patients, because they are in cardiac arrest, receive a full 1.0-mg dose every 3 to 5 minutes.
- **Transcutaneous Cardiac Pacing (TCP)**
  - Cardiac pacing is an equally acceptable alternative to atropine sulfate, especially if you are having difficulty obtaining IV access.
  - Cardiac pacing and administration of atropine can be accomplished simultaneously as well, especially in patients who are profoundly bradycardic.
  - Cardiac pacing can be painful for the patient. Sedation with a benzodiazepine drug (Valium, Versed) may therefore be needed.

Patients with symptomatic bradycardia will typically respond to atropine, unless their bradycardia is not related to excessive parasympathetic stimulation. In these patients, TCP or catecholamines may be the preferred initial intervention.

Other medications used to treat symptomatic bradycardia include dopamine (Intropin) and epinephrine (Adrenalin), both of which are catecholamines and administered as continuous IV infusions. A simple mnemonic to help you remember the recommended order of treatment for a patient with symptomatic bradycardia is "PADE," which stands for **p**acing, **a**tropine, **d**opamine, and **e**pinephrine. We will leave isoproterenol (Isuprel) out of this mnemonic, as it is a last resort drug for symptomatic bradycardia, is potentially harmful to the patient (significantly increases myocardial oxygen demand), and is rarely administered.

Prior to pharmacologic or electrical interventions, and depending on locally established protocols, a fluid bolus of 20 mL/kg may be given in an attempt to raise the patient's blood pressure. If this is considered a viable option, the paramedic must exercise caution, as excess fluids may exacerbate any accompanying pulmonary edema.

As with any patient who presents with cardiac compromise, a 12-lead ECG should be obtained as soon as possible. In the case of this patient, it is clear that his signs and symptoms are related to his bradycardia. However, a 12-lead ECG may reveal other underlying problems, such as myocardial ischemia.

6. Is further treatment required for this patient?

In an attempt to play catch-up with his medications, this patient has effectively depressed his sympathetic nervous system by taking too much of his Lopressor. This would clearly explain his bradycardia and hypotension, both of which have been refractory to previous interventions.

Knowing this important piece of information, you should now administer the most appropriate drug for sympathetic nervous system depression, which is the sympathetic nervous system stimulant, epinephrine. Begin the epinephrine infusion at 2 μg/min, and titrate upward to 10 μg/min, or until the patient's signs and symptoms improve.

7. Are there any special considerations for this patient?

In contrast to those with vagal induced bradycardias, therapeutic effects of epinephrine in its standard dose of 2 to 10 μg/min may not be seen in patients who have overdosed on a beta-blocker, so higher doses may be required in order to achieve hemodynamic stability. In addition, patients with severe overdose may require other medications, such as glucagon, which through its positive inotropic effect, may be useful in increasing blood pressure. IV fluid boluses of up to 1 L may also be required; however, this would not be desirable in the patient with pulmonary edema.

Summary

As we have learned from this case study, bradycardia is not always a parasympathetic nervous system issue. There are multiple causes of bradycardia, which require you to perform a careful and systematic assessment of the patient. The patient in this case study, who overdosed on his beta-blocking medication, could have suffered total cardiovascular collapse and died if his problem were not identified and promptly treated.

You must carefully and systematically assess the patient for serious signs and symptoms that are linked to the bradycardia, which may include chest pain or pressure, shortness of breath, hypotension, altered mental status, and pulmonary edema.

Initial management involves administering 100% supplemental oxygen for the adequately breathing patient or positive pressure ventilatory support for the inadequately breathing patient (slow/fast respirations, reduced tidal volume).

Initial pharmacologic management includes atropine. Transcutaneous pacing can be initiated as well, especially for bradycardias accompanied by AV heart block. If these interventions are unsuccessful, dopamine and epinephrine may be needed. If the underlying cause of the bradycardia can be identified, such as with the patient in this case study, medications that are target-specific (epinephrine for beta-blocker overdose) would be the most appropriate initial therapy.

14

59-Year-Old Female with Abdominal Pain

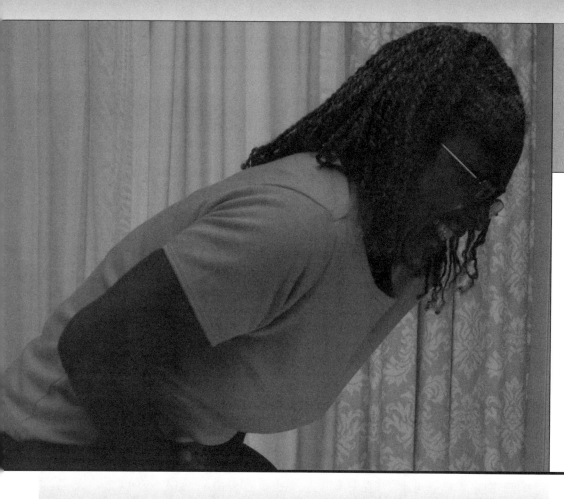

At 10:30 pm, you receive a call to 216 Ivy Ln, Apt 205, for a 59-year-old female with abdominal pain. Your response time to the scene is approximately 10 minutes.

You arrive at the scene at 10:40 pm. A police officer is present to provide assistance. You are escorted to the bedroom by the patient's husband, where you find her doubled over in pain. She is restless and noticeably diaphoretic. You introduce yourself to the patient and perform an initial assessment **(Table 14-1)**. The police officer retrieves the stretcher from the ambulance.

Table 14-1 Initial Assessment

Level of Consciousness	Conscious and alert to person, place, and time, but restless
Chief Complaint	"I have a sharp pain in my abdomen."
Airway and Breathing	Airway patent; respirations, 24 breaths/min with adequate tidal volume
Circulation	Pulse, rapid and weak; skin, cool and diaphoretic

1. What initial management is indicated for this patient?

_____

_____

_____

_____

You perform the appropriate initial management for the patient. The police officer returns with the stretcher, and you place the patient onto it. She immediately lies on her side, and draws her knees into her abdomen. You perform a focused history and physical examination **(Table 14-2)** as your partner obtains additional information from the patient's husband.

Table 14-2 Focused History and Physical Examination

Onset	"This started suddenly, after I returned home from the store."
Provocation/Palliation	"Nothing makes this pain better. It is just as bad now as when it started."
Quality	"It feels like someone is sticking a hot knife into my belly."
Radiation/Referred Pain	"My lower back also hurts."
Severity	"This is the worst pain that I have ever had in my life!"
Time	"This started about 30 minutes ago."
Interventions Prior to EMS Arrival	"I was going to take some Motrin, but we were out."
Abdominal Exam	Tense, no signs of trauma, diffusely tender to palpation
Oxygen Saturation	97% (on 100% oxygen)

As you are retrieving the blood pressure cuff and stethoscope from the jump kit, your partner attaches the ECG leads and obtains a cardiac rhythm tracing **(Figure 14-1)**.

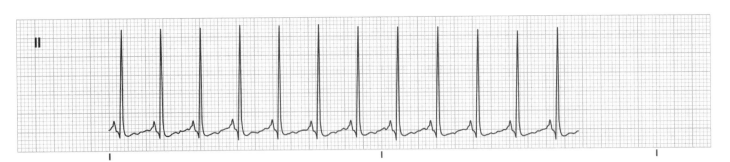

■ **Figure 14-1** Your patient's cardiac rhythm.

2. What is your interpretation of this cardiac rhythm?

_____

_____

_____

Your partner establishes an IV line of normal saline and sets the flow rate to keep the vein open. In the meantime, you obtain baseline vital signs and a SAMPLE history **(Table 14-3)**.

Table 14-3 Baseline Vital Signs and SAMPLE History

Blood Pressure	92/48 mm Hg
Pulse	132 beats/min, weak and regular
Respirations	24 breaths/min, adequate tidal volume
Oxygen Saturation	97% (on 100% oxygen)
Signs and Symptoms	Abdominal pain, hypotension, tachycardia, diaphoresis, weak pulses
Allergies	"I am allergic to sulfa drugs and erythromycin."
Medications	"I take one vitamin per day."
Pertinent Past History	"I am pretty healthy, and do not have any medical problems."
Last Oral Intake	"We ate supper about 4 hours ago."
Events Leading to Present Illness	"I had just returned from the store."

3. What is your field impression of this patient?

_____

_____

_____

4. Are the patient's vital signs and SAMPLE history consistent with your field impression?

_____

_____

_____

On the basis of your field impression of this patient, you establish another IV line of normal saline using a 16-gauge catheter. The patient is quickly but carefully loaded into the ambulance and transported to a trauma center that is approximately 30 miles away.

5. What specific treatment is required for this patient's condition?

_____

_____

_____

En route, the patient remains conscious and alert, though restless. Her pain remains severe, both in her abdomen and her lower back. You quickly perform an ongoing assessment **(Table 14-4)** and then notify the trauma center of your estimated time of arrival, which is approximately 20 minutes.

Table 14-4 Ongoing Assessment

Level of Consciousness	Conscious and alert to person, place, and time, though still restless
Airway and Breathing	Respirations, 24 breaths/min, with adequate tidal volume
Oxygen Saturation	98% (on 100% oxygen)
Blood Pressure	90 mm Hg systolic (by palpation)
Pulse	120 beats/min, weak and regular

6. Is further treatment required for this patient?

_____

_____

_____

_____

7. Are there any special considerations for this patient?

_____

_____

_____

_____

You arrive at the trauma center, where you are met by a team of surgeons. An abdominal computer tomographic (CT) scan reveals a 3-cm dissecting aneurysm, just proximal to the common iliac arteries, in the abdominal aorta. Signs of bleeding are present. The patient is immediately taken to surgery, where the aneurysm is successfully repaired with a Dacron graft. Following a 10-day stay in the hospital, she is discharged home.

CASE STUDY ANSWERS AND SUMMARY

1. What initial management is indicated for this patient?

- **100% supplemental oxygen via nonrebreathing mask**
  - This patient is breathing adequately (adequate tidal volume) and is not in need of positive pressure ventilatory support at this time.
  - Never withhold oxygen from a patient with signs of shock (restlessness, diaphoresis, and tachycardia).

- **Allow a position of comfort**
  - Patients with abdominal pain are typically doubled over or lying on their side with their knees drawn into their chest. This position takes pressure off of the abdominal musculature. Leave them in this position unless it is absolutely necessary to change it.

2. What is your interpretation of this cardiac rhythm?

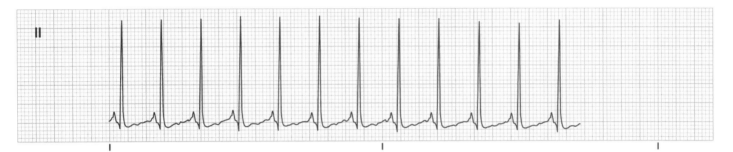

■ **Figure 14-2** Your patient's cardiac rhythm.

This rhythm is a *sinus tachycardia* **(Figure 14-2)**. It is regular, has a ventricular rate of approximately 135 beats/min, and has upright, monomorphic P waves that consistently precede each narrow QRS complex.

Sinus tachycardia is not a treatable rhythm per se, but rather a manifestation of an underlying cause. Common causes of sinus tachycardia include fever, fright, pain, and shock. When a patient is initially seen with sinus tachycardia, you must, through careful and systematic assessment, determine the underlying cause and focus the treatment on that cause. Once the catalyst is removed, the tachycardia will resolve. The tachycardia seen in your patient should be assumed to be the result of shock (hypoperfusion).

3. What is your field impression of this patient?

Although there are numerous causes of acute abdominal pain, in this patient your index of suspicion should be highest for an *abdominal aortic aneurysm (AAA)*. Furthermore, the following assessment findings suggest that the aneurysm is leaking or expanding:

- **The onset of pain** is usually acute and of maximal intensity from the onset. Patients with nonleaking or expanding aortic aneurysms are typically asymptomatic.

- **The quality of the pain** is commonly described as a ripping or tearing sensation, or as though a hot knife has entered the abdomen and exited the lower back.

- **Lower back pain** is frequently associated with an expanding or leaking aortic aneurysm. It may be the primary focal point of the pain or it may radiate from the abdominal or epigastric region.

- **Diffuse abdominal pain** suggests that blood leaking into the abdominal cavity is causing peritoneal irritation.
- **Hypotension, tachycardia, restlessness, and diaphoresis** are all indicative of shock.

An aneurysm is a weakening or abnormal dilation in the wall of an artery and is caused by degenerative changes in the tunica media (middle layer) of the artery. Over time, turbulent blood flow may cause the aneurysm to enlarge through a process called dissection, in which a tear in the tunica intima (inner layer) of the vessel allows blood to leak in between the layers of the arterial wall. This process subsequently weakens the tunica adventitia (outer layer) of the artery.

Abdominal aortic aneurysms affect approximately 2% of the American population. They occur 10 times more commonly in men than in women and are most prevalent in patients between 60 and 70 years of age.

The majority of abdominal aortic aneurysms are caused by destructive changes in the aorta secondary to atherosclerosis or hypertension. Other contributing factors include advanced age, congenital diseases that affect the connective tissue of the blood vessel, and infectious processes such as syphilis (rare). The most common site for an abdominal aortic aneurysm is in the descending aorta, superior to the bifurcation that gives rise to the common iliac arteries. Pulses distal to the aneurysm (femoral, popliteal, and pedal) may be weak or absent. If the aneurysm is confined to one of the common iliac arteries, an ipsilateral pulse deficit may be noted; however, this is less common. When the size of the aneurysm exceeds approximately 4 to 5 cm, it may be palpable as a pulsating mass, located superior to the umbilicus, left of the midline.

Unless the aneurysm begins to expand or leak (dissect), the patient is typically asymptomatic. If, however, dissection occurs, the patient often has a sudden onset of severe pain in the abdomen, epigastrium, or lower back that is frequently described as a ripping or tearing sensation. Signs of shock may also be present as the leaking aneurysm bleeds into the abdominal cavity. The abdomen may be painful to palpation secondary to peritoneal irritation caused by blood.

Acute aortic rupture is characterized by a sudden disappearance of the pulsating mass (if one is present) and profound shock, which is often followed by cardiopulmonary arrest. Approximately 20% of patients with an abdominal aortic aneurysm will suffer acute rupture in the prehospital setting, and roughly 70% to 80% of those patients will die.

4. Are the patient's vital signs and SAMPLE history consistent with your field impression?

The patient's vital signs definitely indicate shock. At present, however, she remains conscious and alert, which indicates adequate cerebral perfusion.

The patient's medical history is essentially unremarkable. None of the typical risk factors for an abdominal aortic aneurysm (hypertension, hyperlipidemia) are present. If she does have hypertension, it has not been diagnosed at this point. It appears as though her age is the only identifiable risk factor.

5. What specific treatment is required for this patient's condition?

The goal in managing a patient with a suspected leaking aortic aneurysm is to take measures in order to prevent acute rupture. Your treatment should be limited to the following:

■ Gentle handling

■ Continued oxygen therapy

■ Two large-bore IV lines of normal saline
  • Set the flow rate to keep the vein open, but be prepared for aggressive fluid resuscitation if signs of aortic rupture occur.

■ Rapid but careful transport with early notification of the receiving hospital
  • Early notification of the receiving hospital is vital so that preparations for immediate surgical intervention can be made.

Hypotension associated with small leaks in the aorta is thought to be secondary to a vasovagal response, rather than internal hemorrhage. Therefore, fluid resuscitation would be less aggressive than in patients with signs of acute aortic rupture.

If signs of rupture occur, rapid fluid resuscitation will clearly be indicated for the patient. On the basis of locally established protocols, the pneumatic antishock garment (PASG) may be used as well. If the PASG is used, inflate both the legs and then the abdominal compartment.

6. Is further treatment required for this patient?

Considering that you suspect a leaking abdominal aortic aneurysm, this patient is *relatively* stable. Further treatment at this point should focus on close, continuous monitoring for signs of aortic rupture. Further palpation of her abdomen would be of no value, as it would only cause unnecessary pain and may precipitate aortic rupture. The IV lines should be maintained at a keep-vein-open rate.

7. Are there any special considerations for this patient?

Patients with aneurysms of the aorta are walking time bombs, and the avoidance of interventions that may precipitate rupture deserves reemphasis. In addition to maintaining the IV lines at a keep-vein-open rate, you should also take measures to minimize the patient's anxiety, which includes allowing the patient to assume a position of comfort, providing reassurance to the patient, and transporting the patient carefully to the hospital.

Summary

Once a patient with an abdominal aortic aneurysm has been identified, treatment will depend on whether or not you suspect that the aneurysm is leaking or expanding, or if acute rupture has occurred.

Management for all patients experiencing an abdominal aortic aneurysm includes ensuring adequate oxygenation and ventilation, initiating two large-bore IV lines, minimizing anxiety, and providing careful transport to the closest appropriate facility for immediate surgical intervention.

If you suspect leakage from the aneurysm, avoid aggressive fluid resuscitation, even if the patient is mildly hypotensive. If signs of rupture occur (profound shock, disappearance of the pulsating mass), aggressive management, including rapid IV fluid administration, possibly use of a PASG, and CPR if the patient is in cardiac arrest, is clearly indicated.

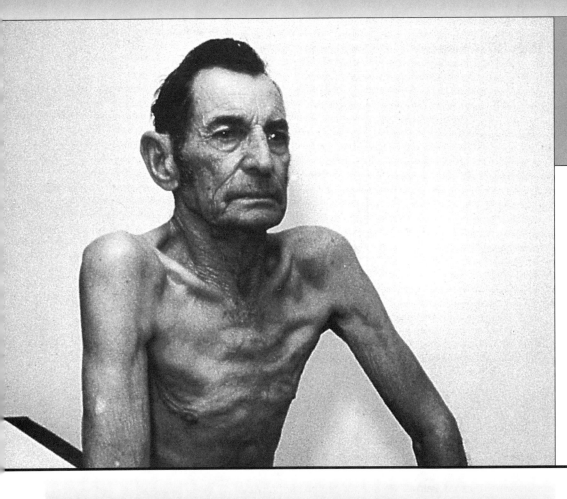

15

62-Year-Old Male in Respiratory Distress

At 11:55 am, your unit is dispatched to a local urgent care clinic at 321 S Main St for a 62-year-old male in respiratory distress. Your response time to the scene is approximately 3 minutes.

You arrive at the clinic at 11:58 and are directed to one of the treatment rooms by a nurse. You find the patient sitting in a tripod position in obvious respiratory distress. You introduce yourself to the patient, who speaks to you in broken sentences. As your partner opens the jump kit, you perform an initial assessment **(Table 15-1)**.

Table 15-1 Initial Assessment

Level of Consciousness	Conscious, but confused
Chief Complaint	The patient is slow to answer questions, and states in broken sentences, "I am having more trouble breathing than I usually do."
Airway and Breathing	Airway patent; respirations, rapid and labored
Circulation	Radial pulse, increased, weak, and irregular; perioral cyanosis present

The clinic nurse tells you that she attempted to place the patient on oxygen, but he kept removing the mask from his face. She tried applying a nasal cannula, which the patient also refused.

1. What initial management is indicated for this patient?

_____

_____

_____

_____

With the assistance of the clinic nurse, your partner initiates the appropriate airway management. The nurse tells you that the patient's condition has worsened since he first arrived at the clinic. She provides you with his presenting information as you perform a focused history and physical examination **(Table 15-2)**.

Table 15-2 Focused History and Physical Examination

Onset	"The patient told me that he recently had 'flu-like symptoms', which were followed by a sudden worsening of the respiratory distress that he normally has."
Provocation/Palliation	"He said that it was a little easier to breathe when he leans forward."
Quality	"He was able to speak in full sentences initially, but now he can barely get two words out."
Radiation/Referred Pain	"He did not complain of any pain."
Severity	"Compared to his initial presentation, his breathing is much worse now."
Time	"He told me that this began yesterday afternoon."
Interventions Prior to EMS Arrival	"I tried to give him oxygen, but he would not allow it, either by face mask or nasal cannula."
Chest Exam	Chest is barrel-shaped; intercostal retractions and use of accessory muscles are noted.
Breath Sounds	Breath sounds are diminished bilaterally; expiratory wheezing and rhonchi are heard in all lung fields.
Oxygen Saturation	83% (ventilated with 100% oxygen)
Temperature	101.5° F

The patient was placed on a cardiac monitor prior to your arrival. You run a 6-second strip and analyze his cardiac rhythm **(Figure 15-1)**.

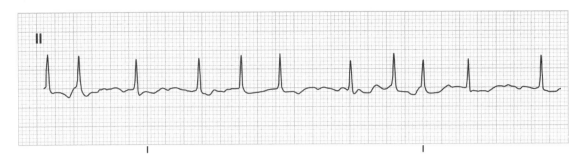

■ **Figure 15-1** Your patient's cardiac rhythm.

2. What is your interpretation of this cardiac rhythm?

You obtain baseline vital signs and a SAMPLE history **(Table 15-3)**. A receptionist hands you the patient's medical records, from which you obtain his medical history.

Table 15-3 Baseline Vital Signs and SAMPLE History

Blood Pressure	148/88 mm Hg
Pulse	110 beats/min, weak and irregular
Respirations	32 breaths/min, labored (baseline); ventilation rate, 15 breaths/min
Oxygen Saturation	81% (ventilated with 100% oxygen)
Signs and Symptoms	Recent cold symptoms, severe respiratory distress, retractions, cyanosis, confusion
Allergies	Penicillin, aspirin, Demerol
Medications	Albuterol, Lanoxin, warfarin, Aldomet
Pertinent Past History	Emphysema, hypertension, atrial fibrillation, long history of smoking
Last Oral Intake	According to the nurse, "His last meal was the previous night. He could not remember the exact time."
Events Leading to Present Illness	Recent cold symptoms

3. What is your field impression of this patient?

_____

_____

_____

_____

As your partner continues to manage the patient's airway, you quickly establish an IV line of normal saline and set the flow rate to keep the vein open.

4. Are the patient's vital signs and SAMPLE history consistent with your field impression?

_____

_____

_____

_____

Despite positive pressure ventilation with the bag-valve-mask (BVM) device, the patient's oxygen saturation continues to fall. Additionally, his mental status has markedly diminished. Your partner states that he is meeting significant resistance when ventilating.

5. What specific treatment is required for this patient's condition?

_____

_____

_____

_____

Your partner has definitively secured the patient's airway, and the appropriate medications have been administered. Following these interventions, a quick reassessment of the patient shows marked improvement in oxygen saturation. You place him onto the stretcher, load him into the ambulance, and begin transport to a hospital that is 7 miles away. En route, you connect the patient to an automatic transport ventilator (ATV), perform an ongoing assessment **(Table 15-4)**, and then call your radio report to the receiving hospital.

Table 15-4 Ongoing Assessment

Level of Consciousness	Improved, becoming resistant to ventilatory support
Airway and Breathing	Intubated and ventilated at a rate of 15 breaths/min
Oxygen Saturation	92% (ventilated with 100% oxygen)
Blood Pressure	138/80 mm Hg
Pulse	96 beats/min, strong and irregular
Chest Exam	Minimal intercostal retractions
Breath Sounds	Widespread rales and a few wheezes, otherwise equal bilaterally

6. Is further treatment required for this patient?

7. Are there any special considerations for this patient?

The patient is delivered to the emergency department. His condition has improved significantly following your treatment. You give your verbal report to the attending physician, who orders a stat portable chest radiograph and an arterial blood gas analysis.

Following additional assessment and management in the emergency department, the patient is diagnosed with acute chronic obstructive pulmonary disease (COPD) exacerbation secondary to pneumonia.

He is given additional medications, including antibiotics, and is admitted to the medical intensive care unit. Following a 10-day stay in the hospital, the patient is discharged home.

1. What initial management is indicated for this patient?

- **Positive pressure ventilations (bag-valve-mask device or pocket-mask device)**
  - This patient has multiple signs of inadequate breathing, including confusion, rapid and labored respirations, inability to speak in full sentences, and perioral cyanosis.
  - Tidal volume is needed and can only be provided with the use of positive pressure ventilatory support.
  - Consider placing a nasopharyngeal airway if the patient's level of consciousness further decreases.

2. What is your interpretation of this cardiac rhythm?

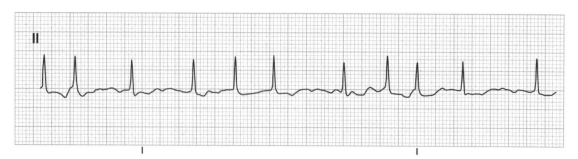

■ **Figure 15-2** Your patient's cardiac rhythm.

The cardiac rhythm depicted is *atrial fibrillation,* which is characterized by an irregularly irregular rhythm and the absence of discernable P waves **(Figure 15-2)**.

Atrial fibrillation is caused by multiple ectopic foci in the atria that discharge in a chaotic fashion. Many of the impulses are blocked at the AV junction, while others are allowed to pass through to the ventricles. This randomized impulse passage through the AV junction causes the ventricular rhythm in atrial fibrillation to be irregularly irregular.

Atrial fibrillation is often seen with conditions such as congestive heart failure and COPD (eg, emphysema) and is commonly caused by pulmonary hypertension with subsequent atrial dilation.

3. What is your field impression of this patient?

This patient is suffering from an *acute exacerbation of emphysema* and is quickly approaching complete respiratory failure. The following assessment findings support this field impression:

- **History of emphysema,** no doubt attributed to his history of cigarette smoking, is characterized by the barrel-shaped appearance of his chest.
- **Recent flu-like symptoms,** which indicate a possible respiratory tract infection, the most common precursor to acute exacerbation of COPD.
- **Temperature of 101.5° F,** which confirms the presence of an infection.
- **Acute worsening of his shortness of breath,** which is classic in COPD exacerbation following an acute respiratory tract infection.

Emphysema falls within a myriad of conditions collectively called COPD. Other forms of COPD include chronic bronchitis, and, to a lesser degree, asthma, which is more of an episodic disease rather than a chronic one.

Emphysema is a progressive, irreversible pulmonary disease that is most often attributed to a history of long-term cigarette smoking or repeated exposure to other toxic substances. The incidence of emphysema is much higher in men than in women.

Emphysema results in gradual destruction of the alveolar walls due to a loss of pulmonary surfactant, which decreases the surface area of the alveolar membrane and interferes with gas exchange in the lungs. Additionally, the number of pulmonary capillaries decreases, which increases the resistance to pulmonary blood flow. This process ultimately causes pulmonary hypertension, which may lead to right-sided heart failure (cor pulmonale). Because the right side of the heart must pump against a high-pressure gradient, atrial dilation may occur, thus resulting in atrial fibrillation.

Emphysema also weakens the walls of the small bronchioles, which, in combination with alveolar wall destruction, decreases the ability of the lungs to effectively recoil during exhalation. This causes air to become trapped in the lungs, giving the person's chest a characteristic barrel-shaped appearance. Frequent pulmonary infections further the degree of air trapping because of inflammation and mucous production within the bronchioles **(Figure 15-3)**.

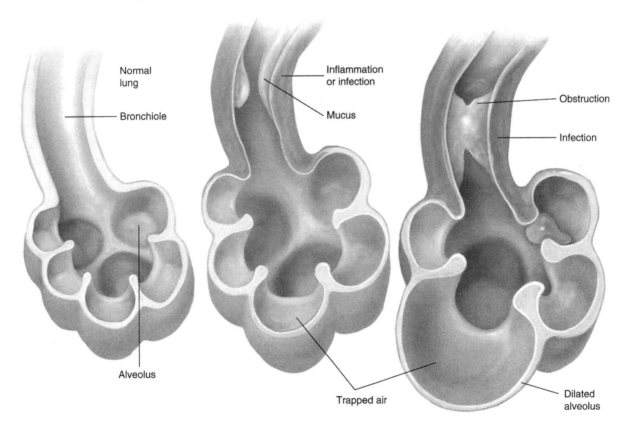

■ **Figure 15-3** Pulmonary infections in already damaged airwaves.

The destruction of lung tissue causes the alveoli to collapse (atelectasis). The patient attempts to compensate for this by breathing through pursed lips, thus creating an effect similar to that of positive-end expiratory pressure (PEEP).

As the degenerative process of emphysema continues, the partial pressure of oxygen in the arterial blood (PaO_2) decreases and remains chronically low. This stimulates red blood cell production, perhaps even to excessive levels (polycythemia), which would explain why the patient's skin remains pink (pink puffer) despite inadequate pulmonary gas exchange. The presence of cyanosis, therefore, would indicate severe hypoxia in patients with emphysema, more so than if it were present in an otherwise healthy person.

Patients with COPD tend to retain carbon dioxide and, therefore, have a chronically elevated partial pressure of arterial carbon dioxide ($PaCO_2$). Chemoreceptors that monitor the levels of oxygen in carbon dioxide in the body eventually become accustomed to this, and the respiratory center in the brain (medulla oblongata) stops using increased $PaCO_2$ levels to regulate breathing, as it does in an otherwise healthy person. This activates a mechanism called the hypoxic drive, which increases breathing stimulation when PaO_2 levels fall and inhibits breathing stimulation when PaO_2 levels increase. In rare cases, the administration of high-concentration oxygen, which can quickly increase PaO_2 levels, may cause the chemoreceptors to stop stimulating the respiratory centers, resulting in hypoventilation or even apnea. If this occurs, simply assist the patient's ventilations. Never withhold oxygen from a hypoxic patient, even in the face of this potential, although highly uncommon, threat.

Patients with emphysema are predisposed to lower respiratory tract infections such as pneumonia because of their diminished ability to effectively expel secretions from the lungs. In addition, hypoxia-related cardiac dysrhythmias may occur.

Patients with emphysema and COPD in general learn to live with their chronic illness on a daily basis and grow accustomed to the normal respiratory distress and physical limitations that accompany it. When they call EMS, something has changed for the worst.

The signs and symptoms of emphysema are summarized in **Table 15-5**.

Table 15-5 Signs and Symptoms of Emphysema

Barrel-chest appearance
Nonproductive cough
Severe exertional dyspnea
Pink skin color
Wheezing and rhonchi
Pursed-lip breathing (prolonged inspiration)

4. Are the patient's vital signs and SAMPLE history consistent with your field impression?

The patient's vital signs do not reinforce a field impression of COPD exacerbation as much as his medical history does. In particular, the recent flu-like symptoms that preceded an acute exacerbation of his respiratory distress make this a classic case.

Because this patient takes numerous medications, each of which is used to treat different conditions, it would be worthwhile to briefly review each of them.

- **Albuterol (Ventolin, Proventil)**
  - Selective beta$_2$-agonist that dilates the bronchioles and is thus used to treat diseases associated with bronchiole constriction and/or inflammation, such as asthma, emphysema, and bronchitis

- **Lanoxin (Digoxin, Digitalis)**
  - A cardiac glycoside that is used for, among other conditions, ventricular rate control in patients with chronic atrial fibrillation

- **Warfarin (Coumadin)**
  - An anticoagulant commonly prescribed as prophylactic therapy to patients with atrial fibrillation who are prone to developing microemboli (small clots) when blood stagnates in the poorly contracting atria

- Methyldopa (Aldomet)
  - A centrally acting antiadrenergic used in the treatment of hypertension. Its active metabolite, alpha-methylnorepinephrine, lowers the blood pressure by stimulating central inhibitory alpha-adrenergic receptors and reducing plasma levels of renin. Renin is a proteolytic enzyme of the kidney that plays a major role in the release of angiotensin, a potent vasoconstrictor.

5. What specific treatment is required for this patient's condition?

- Endotracheal intubation
  - If the paramedic has difficulty providing effective ventilations utilizing basic means (bag-valve-mask device, pocket-mask device), endotracheal intubation should be performed to facilitate administration of 100% oxygen directly into the patient's lungs and more definitively protect the patient's airway.
  - As evidenced by the patient's falling oxygen saturation level and markedly diminished level of consciousness, it is clear that bag-valve-mask ventilation is not providing adequate oxygenation.
  - Because of the patient's already diminished level of consciousness, a hypnotic-sedative drug (Versed, Etomidate) may be all that is required in order to facilitate intubation. If, however, sedation alone is not effective, a neuromuscular blocker (paralytic) may be needed to perform rapid sequence intubation (RSI).
    - When inducing paralysis with medications, succinylcholine (Anectine) is the preferred initial agent to use. Succinylcholine has a duration of action of only 3 to 5 minutes, which means that if intubation is unsuccessful, you will not have to ventilate the patient with a BVM device for a prolonged period of time. Succinylcholine does, however, depolarize potassium ions, which produces muscular fasciculations (generalized muscle twitching). Therefore, use of a nondepolarizing paralytic, such as vecuronium (Norcuron) in a premedication, or priming, dose prior to inducing full neuromuscular blockade with succinylcholine is advisable. Once intubation is *successfully performed and confirmed*, neuromuscular blockade can be maintained with a longer-acting paralytic, especially if your transport time is going to be prolonged. Again, vecuronium, which has a 45-minute duration of action, would be an appropriate drug to use.
    - Follow locally established protocols regarding the use and doses of neuromuscular blockers for RSI.
- Pharmacologic interventions
  - *Aerosolized bronchodilators* can be administered endotracheally with a small-volume inline nebulizer. The following medications can be given alone, or in combination:
    - Selective beta$_2$-adrenergic agonists, such as albuterol (Ventolin, Proventil), metaproterenol (Alupent), or isoetharine (Bronkosol)
    - Anticholinergic bronchodilators such as ipratropium (Atrovent)
      - When used in combination with beta$_2$ agonists, the beta$_2$ agonist must be administered first, followed by a 5-minute interval prior to administering Atrovent.

Aerosolized bronchodilators, because of their rapid onset of action (3 to 5 minutes), would be the preferred initial pharmacologic intervention because of the severity of the patient's condition. The significant bronchoconstriction, which is impairing effective positive pressure ventilation in this patient, must be reversed as soon as possible. Follow locally established protocols regarding the dose of endotracheally administered bronchodilators.

- *Intravenous glucosteroids*
  - Methylprednisolone (Solu-Medrol): Reduces acute and chronic inflammation and potentiates the relaxation of bronchiole smooth muscle caused by beta-adrenergic agonists.
    - Solu-Medrol has an onset of action of approximately 1 to 2 hours. The adult dose varies, and usually ranges from 40 to 125 mg IV.

The goal in treating patients with acute COPD decompensation — or any lower airway disorder for that matter — is to correct hypoxemia and to relieve the bronchoconstriction that is causing the hypoxemia. These actions will prevent respiratory failure and subsequent cardiac arrest.

Administration of 100% supplemental oxygen is the first and most important intervention. Oxygen may be given with a nonrebreathing mask or via positive pressure ventilatory support if the patient's respiratory effort is inadequate.

Medications, administered either by aerosol or IV or both, are needed to relax the smooth muscles of the lower airways, thus improving ventilation and facilitating oxygenation.

6. Is further treatment required for this patient?

By improving this patient's oxygenation status, his level of consciousness has improved, and he is now resisting the endotracheal tube. Because of the potential for vomiting and aspiration following removal of the endotracheal tube and the possibility that his condition could worsen, he should remain intubated. Extubation in the field (unless done by the patient) is not commonly performed. For patient comfort and to prevent field extubation by the patient, consider administering additional doses of a long-acting paralytic (eg, Norcuron) and/or keep the patient sedated with the appropriate medications (Versed, Valium).

Although his oxygen saturation of 92% is slightly low, it may be as good as it gets for this chronically ill patient, and is still better than 81%! Continue to monitor his ventilatory status, oxygen saturation, and electrocardiogram. He is still prone to cardiac dysrhythmias.

7. Are there any special considerations for this patient?

As previously mentioned, patients with COPD have chronically low PaO_2 levels and are occasionally stimulated to breathe based on these levels (hypoxic drive).

If high concentrations of oxygen are administered, the respiratory centers in the brain may be fooled into thinking that the patient is adequately oxygenated and will therefore send messages to the respiratory muscles to decrease the rate and strength of breathing. Oxygen-induced hypoventilation or apnea occurs in less than 3% to 5% of patients with COPD. Should this rare event occur, simply provide positive pressure ventilatory support. Never withhold oxygen from a hypoxic patient!

Summary

When patients with chronic respiratory disease call EMS, a significant change has occurred in their condition. Otherwise your assistance would not have been requested.

Due to the nature of their illness, patients with COPD typically have a baseline respiratory distress; however, they cannot live with *severe* hypoxia any better than a healthy person would.

An acute lower respiratory tract infection, such as pneumonia, in which the patient cannot effectively expel secretions from their lungs, is the most common precursor to exacerbation of COPD. The mucous production and bronchiole inflammation that accompany many respiratory infections only worsen the patient's hypoxia.

You must perform a careful, systematic assessment of the patient and provide the appropriate treatment in a timely manner. It is critical that you recognize the difference between an adequately and inadequately breathing patient.

Prehospital care focuses on ensuring adequate oxygenation and ventilation and pharmacologically reversing bronchoconstriction. Definitive care includes treating the underlying cause of the exacerbation, which usually involves antibiotics to treat the underlying infection. If the patient begins to show signs of respiratory failure, such as a rapidly falling oxygen saturation level or decreasing level of consciousness, use sedating agents and neuromuscular blocking medications to intubate the patient without delay.

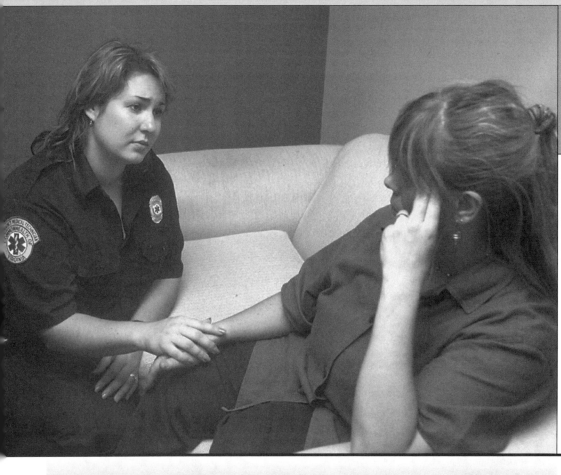

16

29-Year-Old Female with Anxiety and Palpitations

The time is 10:11 am. Your unit is dispatched to 111 Arkansas Pass for a 29-year-old female who is experiencing anxiety and palpitations. Your response time to the scene is approximately 9 minutes.

You arrive at the scene at 10:20 am and are met at the door by the patient. She is crying and noticeably shaking. You sit her down on the sofa in her living room and perform an initial assessment (Table 16-1).

Table 16-1 Initial Assessment

Level of Consciousness	Conscious and alert to person, place, and time, crying
Chief Complaint	"I feel like I'm going to die! My hands and face are numb, and my heart is racing."
Airway and Breathing	Airway is patent; respirations are rapid, with adequate depth
Circulation	Radial pulse is rapid, strong, and regular; skin is diaphoretic

1. What initial management is indicated for this patient?

_____

_____

_____

_____

Following the appropriate intervention, the patient is now breathing at 24 breaths/min with adequate depth. The pulse oximeter reads 98% on room air. Your partner attempts to administer supplemental oxygen, but the patient states that it feels like the oxygen mask is smothering her. You perform a focused history and physical examination **(Table 16-2)** as your partner attaches the ECG leads to the patient's chest.

Table 16-2 Focused History and Physical Examination

Onset	"This began suddenly."
Provocation/Palliation	"I was in a state of panic, and could not control my breathing. I felt like I was going to die."
Quality	"It felt like I was smothering."
Radiation/Referred Pain	"I had a sharp pain in the middle of my chest, which is better now. The pain stayed in my chest."
Time	"This began about 20 minutes ago."
Interventions Prior to EMS Arrival	None
Breath Sounds	Breath sounds are clear and equal bilaterally.
Oxygen Saturation	99% (on room air).
Blood Glucose	102 mg/dL
Pupils	Equal and reactive to light

A 6-second strip of the patient's cardiac rhythm is obtained **(Figure 16-1)**. As you are analyzing the cardiac rhythm, the patient, who is still crying, says that she feels like she's "losing it."

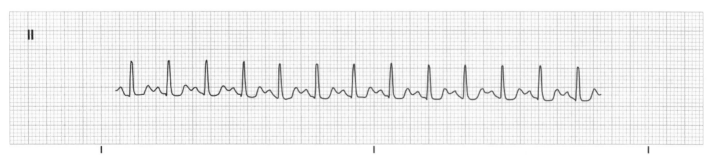

■ **Figure 16-1** Your patient's cardiac rhythm.

2. What is your interpretation of this cardiac rhythm?

_____

_____

_____

_____

The patient is continuing to cry and is still having tremors. She fears that she will have another attack. Your partner attempts to provide emotional support and reassurance as you obtain baseline vital signs and a SAMPLE history **(Table 16-3)**.

Table 16-3 Baseline Vital Signs and SAMPLE History

Blood Pressure	156/92 mm Hg
Pulse	148 beats/min, strong and regular
Respirations	22 breaths/min, adequate depth
Oxygen Saturation	99% (on room air)
Signs and Symptoms	Hyperventilation (resolved), carpopedal spasm (resolved), tachycardia, emotional upset, tremors
Allergies	"I am not allergic to any medications."
Medications	Xanax, Prozac
Pertinent Past History	"I am being treated for anxiety and depression"
Last Oral Intake	"I haven't eaten since last night. I was too nervous to eat today."
Events Leading to Present Illness	"I wasn't doing anything. This just came on suddenly and unexpectedly. I have been taking my medications as prescribed. Aren't they supposed to prevent this?"

3. What is your field impression of this patient?

_____

_____

_____

_____

4. Are the patient's vital signs and SAMPLE history consistent with your field impression?

_____

_____

_____

_____

The patient's respirations remain under control, and she is now gaining feeling back in her face and hands. She is, however, still emotionally upset and crying. Her heart rate remains elevated, and she is still diaphoretic. The patient asks you to take her to the hospital because she is afraid to stay at home by herself. However, she refuses to allow you to start an IV line.

5. What specific treatment is required for this patient's condition?

_____

_____

_____

_____

On her own accord, the patient walks to the ambulance. You administer the appropriate intervention to provide symptomatic relief for the patient, and then initiate transport her to the hospital, which is approximately 25 miles away. En route, you conduct an ongoing assessment **(Table 16-4)**, and then call your radio report to the receiving hospital.

Table 16-4 Ongoing Assessment

Level of Consciousness	Conscious and alert to person, place, and time; drowsy
Airway and Breathing	Respirations are 14 breaths/min, adequate depth
Oxygen Saturation	99% (on room air)
Blood Pressure	136/84 mm Hg
Pulse	78 beats/min, strong and regular
Breath Sounds	Clear and equal bilaterally
Pupils	Equal and reactive to light

The patient continues to improve en route. She tells you that the numbness in her face and hands has fully resolved. Her cardiac rhythm has improved as well **(Figure 16-2)**.

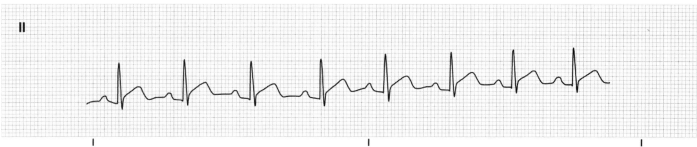

■ **Figure 16-2** Your patient's cardiac rhythm has improved.

6. Is further treatment required for this patient?

_____

_____

_____

7. Are there any special considerations for this patient?

_____

_____

_____

The patient is delivered to the emergency department. Her symptoms have resolved, and she remains somewhat drowsy because of the treatment that you provided.

You give your verbal report to the charge nurse. Following a 12-lead ECG, which was unremarkable, and an arterial blood gas analysis, which gave normal results, the patient is discharged home. She is told to follow up with her physician for a possible adjustment in her prescribed medications.

CASE STUDY ANSWERS AND SUMMARY

1. What initial management is indicated for this patient?

- **Reassurance and respiratory coaching**
  - Instruct the patient to attempt to reduce the rate and depth of her respirations, and provide emotional support and reassurance throughout this process.

Perform a careful assessment, monitor the patient's oxygen saturation, and give supplemental oxygen if necessary. Be prepared to assist ventilations if the patient's tidal volume becomes markedly reduced (shallow breathing) or her level of consciousness decreases.

Hyperventilation syndrome, although most commonly caused by excessive anxiety, can also result from other conditions, many of which are life-threatening **(Table 16-5)**.

Table 16-5 Nonanxiety Causes of Hyperventilation Syndrome
Metabolic acidosis
• Diabetic ketoacidosis
• Aspirin (salicylate) overdose
Central nervous system disorders
• Hemorrhagic stroke
• Space-occupying intracranial lesions (tumors)
Hypoxia from any cause
Acute myocardial infarction
Acute respiratory conditions
• Pulmonary embolism
• Asthma
• Congestive heart failure
• Pneumonia
Severe pain or fever

Do not attempt to increase the patient's PCO_2 level by having her breathe into a paper bag or applying an oxygen mask without oxygen flowing. These interventions are no longer recommended and could be lethal if the hyperventilation is not related to anxiety.

2. What is your interpretation of this cardiac rhythm?

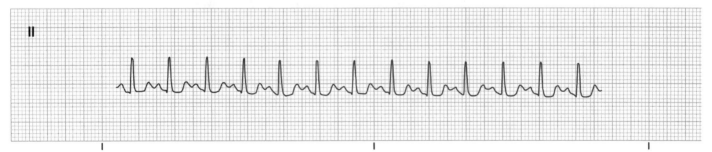

■ **Figure 16-3** Your patient's cardiac rhythm.

This patient's cardiac rhythm is a *sinus tachycardia* **(Figure 16-3)**. The rhythm is regular, has a ventricular rate of approximately 145 beats/min, and has narrow QRS complexes that are all consistently preceded by monomorphic P waves.

In this particular patient, sinus tachycardia is most likely attributed to an anxiety-induced sympathetic nervous system discharge of epinephrine. A careful assessment, however, is still required in order to rule out more serious causes (eg, hypoxia).

3. What is your field impression of this patient?

It is clear that this patient is having an anxiety (panic) attack. The following assessment findings support this field impression:

- **Hyperventilation**, which your partner was able to correct by providing reassurance and coaching of the patient's respirations. Hypoxia-related hyperventilation typically does not respond to coaching and emotional reassurance. If left untreated, hyperventilation may result in respiratory alkalosis due to elimination of excess carbon dioxide and possibly metabolic alkalosis (increased blood pH) due to excess excretion of hydrogen ions (H+).

- **Carpopedal spasm**, which is secondary to the hyperventilation, results from excessive CO_2 elimination and an increased amount of bound calcium (relative hypocalcemia).

- **Signs of excessive anxiety**, such as tremors, tachycardia, crying, and a feeling of "losing it."

An anxiety (panic) attack can be a terrifying ordeal for the patient, and, from a management standpoint, a dilemma for the paramedic. *The Diagnostic and Statistical Manual of Mental Disorders,* 4th edition text revised *(DSM-IV-TR),* which is published by the American Psychiatric Association, does not classify a panic attack as a disease, but rather an event that falls within a broad category referred to as Generalized Anxiety Disorder, or GAD **(Table 16-6)**. GAD is defined as excessive anxiety and recurrent worrying that persists for at least 6 months.

Table 16-6 Generalized Anxiety Disorder

Restlessness or feeling "on the edge"
Easily fatigued
Difficulty concentrating
Irritability
Muscle tension
Sleep disturbances

A diagnosis of GAD is typically made if the patient has at least three of the signs and symptoms listed in Table 16-6 that persist for at least 6 months, occurring on more days than not.

Panic disorder falls within the category of GAD, as do phobic (fear) disorders and posttraumatic stress disorder.

A panic attack, also commonly referred to as an anxiety attack, begins acutely, and is generally unprovoked. The signs and symptoms **(Table 16-7)** typically peak within the first 10 minutes following the onset and generally subside in less than 1 hour.

Table 16-7 Signs and Symptoms of a Panic Attack

Hyperventilation
Carpopedal spasm
• Numbness, tingling, and spasms of the hands and feet
Tachycardia or palpitations
Tremors
Nausea
Diaphoresis
Chest pain or discomfort
Dizziness or light-headedness
Fear of dying, losing control, or going crazy

If the patient has an established history of an anxiety disorder and is of an age where cardiac or pulmonary disease is less commonly seen, a panic attack is the most likely cause. A careful and systematic assessment of the patient is still required, however, because young people do experience acute myocardial infarctions, strokes, and other serious conditions, although much less often. A field impression of panic attack is made by a process of elimination.

4. Are the patient's vital signs and SAMPLE history consistent with your field impression?

This patient's vital signs indicate a sympathetic nervous system discharge of epinephrine, which is causing her tachycardia and hypertension.

Her medical history is consistent with GAD. She also has depression, which commonly accompanies GAD.

The sudden, unprovoked onset of her symptoms is consistent with a panic attack. The following prescribed medications are used to treat her condition:

■ **Aprazolam (Xanax)** is a benzodiazepine used in the treatment of chronic anxiety because of its anxiolytic effects.

■ **Fluoxetine (Prozac)** is a selective serotonin-reuptake inhibitor (SSRI) used to treat, among other conditions, depression and obsessive-compulsive disorder (OCD).

5. What specific treatment is required for this patient's condition?

Managing a patient with an anxiety disorder is essentially supportive and consists of providing emotional reassurance, and, if needed, administering an anxiolytic medication in order to provide the patient symptomatic relief. Either of the following medications, both of which are benzodiazepine anxiolytics, could be administered to this patient:

■ **Lorazepam (Ativan)** 1 to 4 mg via intramuscular injection. This dose may be repeated in 15 to 20 minutes up to a maximum dose of 8 mg.

■ **Diazepam (Valium)** 5 mg via intramuscular injection, up to 10 mg. Additional dosing may be repeated in 10 to 15 minutes, up to a maximum dose of 30 mg.

Since the patient will not allow you to start an IV line, intramuscular injection is the only route available to administer these drugs. The onset of action when given intramuscularly is typically 15 to 30 minutes, compared to 1 to 5 minutes when given IV.

If a benzodiazepine is administered, you must monitor the patient for signs of CNS depression (hypoventilation, bradycardia, hypotension), which benzodiazepines can propagate.

6. Is further treatment required for this patient?

With continued resolution of the patient's symptoms, additional care should consist of continued emotional reassurance and monitoring for benzodiazepine-induced CNS depression. The drowsiness that she is experiencing is no doubt attributed to the anxiolytic medication she was administered.

7. Are there any special considerations for this patient?

Some patients, in a desperate attempt to stop their panic attack, will take their anxiolytic medications in a higher dose than prescribed, causing CNS depression and death due to respiratory arrest. Your patient claims to be taking the appropriate dosage.

Patients with a history of depression should be considered at risk for suicide. During the course of your assessment and treatment, you should inquire as to whether the patient is having suicidal thoughts, especially since she has medication (Xanax, Prozac) that can be taken in overdose. In contrast to men, who typically commit suicide by more violent means (gunshot wounds), women typically use less violent means, such as overdosing on medications.

Summary

GAD is an empiric psychological disorder that includes a variety of conditions, including phobic disorders, panic disorder, and posttraumatic stress disorder. The paramedic should refer to the *DSM-IV-TR* for more information regarding GAD and panic attacks.

A panic attack is a terrifying event for the patient and can present a management dilemma for the paramedic. Hyperventilation is the most common presentation of a panic attack, which the paramedic must treat carefully. Treatment begins by ruling out life-threatening causes *first,* providing respiratory coaching and reassurance, and administering supplemental oxygen if needed. Some patients will hyperventilate to a point where their tidal volume becomes markedly reduced and may thus require positive pressure ventilatory support.

Anxiolytic medications, such as Valium or Ativan, may be required to provide the patient relief from symptoms.

Remember, the field impression of a panic attack and hyperventilation syndrome should be arrived at through a process of eliminating potentially life-threatening causes. If you are in doubt, provide 100% oxygen, and promptly transport the patient to the hospital.

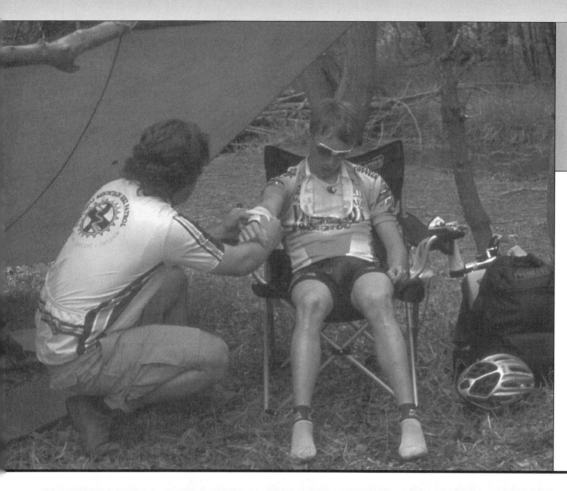

17

23-Year-Old Male with Confusion and Slurred Speech

You and your partner are standing by at a local bike-a-thon. At 1:20 pm, you are approached by a 23-year-old biker who says that he feels like he is going to faint. The temperature outside is 99° F and the relative humidity is 90%.

As your partner starts the ambulance and turns on the air conditioner, you sit the patient down in a chair in the shade. He is confused, his speech is slurred, and his skin is flushed, hot, and diaphoretic. You perform an initial assessment **(Table 17-1)** as your partner brings the jump kit from the ambulance.

Table 17-1 Initial Assessment

Level of Consciousness	Confused, slurred speech
Chief Complaint	"I feel like I am going to faint, and I am nauseated."
Airway and Breathing	Airway, patent; respirations, rapid and deep
Circulation	Radial pulse, rapid and full; skin is flushed, hot, and diaphoretic

1. What initial management is indicated for this patient?

_____

_____

_____

_____

After moving the patient to the back of the cooled ambulance, you perform the appropriate initial management. The patient remains conscious, but confused. Your partner, who has prepared for additional interventions, attaches the ECG leads to the patient's chest. You perform a focused history and physical examination **(Table 17-2)**.

Table 17-2 Focused History and Physical Examination

Source	Exposed to high ambient temperature
Environment	Outside temperature, 99° F; relative humidity, 90%
Duration	"I have been outside for the past 5 hours."
Loss of Consciousness	"No, but I feel like I am going to faint."
Effects	The patient is confused. His skin is flushed, hot, and diaphoretic.
General or Local	Systemic (general) exposure
Temperature	104.8° F

A 6-second strip of the patient's cardiac rhythm has been obtained **(Figure 17-1)**. As you are analyzing the rhythm, your partner obtains personal information (name, date of birth) from the patient.

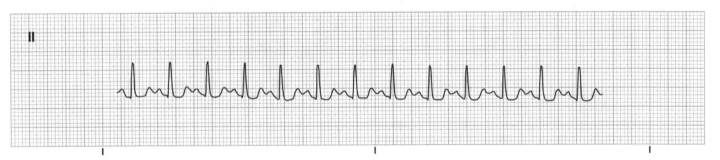

■ **Figure 17-1** Your patient's cardiac rhythm.

2. What is your interpretation of this cardiac rhythm?

_____

_____

_____

_____

The patient's mental status has diminished further. His skin remains hot, flushed, and diaphoretic. You obtain baseline vital signs and a SAMPLE history **(Table 17-3)**; however, the patient is having difficulty answering your questions. You tell your partner to proceed to the hospital immediately.

Table 17-3 Baseline Vital Signs and SAMPLE History

Blood Pressure	88/60 mm Hg
Pulse	144 beats/min, weak and regular
Respirations	28 breaths/min and deep
Oxygen Saturation	98% (on 100% oxygen)
Signs and Symptoms	Confusion, hot and flushed skin, diaphoresis, near syncope, tachycardia, hypotension
Allergies	"I don't think that I am allergic to anything."
Medications	"I don't think so."
Pertinent Past History	"I cannot remember."
Last Oral Intake	"I cannot remember."
Events Leading to Present Illness	"The last thing I remember was getting my bike from the back of my truck."

3. What is your field impression of this patient?

_____

_____

_____

_____

4. Are the patient's vital signs and SAMPLE history consistent with your field impression?

_____

_____

_____

_____

As you proceed to the hospital, which is 20 miles away, you quickly reassess the patient. His mental status has markedly diminished, and his respirations remain increased and deep. Recognizing the seriousness of the patient's condition, you prepare for aggressive treatment.

5. What specific treatment is required for this patient's condition?

_____

_____

_____

_____

While en route to the hospital, you perform interventions aimed at rapidly lowering the patient's core body temperature and replacing lost fluid volume. The patient's mental status is unchanged, and his respirations remain increased and deep. With an estimated time of arrival at the hospital of approximately 15 minutes, you quickly perform an ongoing assessment **(Table 17-4)** and then alert the receiving hospital.

Table 17-4 Ongoing Assessment

Level of Consciousness	Responsive to painful stimuli
Airway and Breathing	Respirations, 28 breaths/min and deep
Oxygen Saturation	98% (on 100% oxygen)
Blood Pressure	110/60 mm Hg
Pulse	118 beats/min, weak and regular
Temperature	102.9° F

6. Is further treatment required for this patient?

_____

_____

_____

_____

Following continued aggressive treatment of this patient, you note improvement in his mental status. His airway remains patent, and his respirations have decreased and are of normal depth. The hospital staff is aware of your impending arrival.

7. Are there any special considerations for this patient?

_____

_____

_____

_____

Upon arriving at the hospital, the attending physician opens the back doors of the ambulance. You give the physician your verbal report as you are moving the patient into the emergency department.

Aggressive treatment is continued in the emergency department. The patient's condition continues to improve, and his core body temperature is now 101.4° F. Blood chemistry analysis reveals derangements in the patient's sodium and potassium levels.

Following additional stabilization in the emergency department, the patient is admitted to the medical intensive care unit. He was discharged home 1 week later without neurologic deficit.

CASE STUDY ANSWERS AND SUMMARY

1. What initial management is indicated for this patient?

■ **Prevent further heat loss**
  - You must immediately remove this patient from the hot environment by moving him to a shady, cooler area or better yet, the back of the ambulance with the air conditioner turned on.
  - Removing excessive clothing will facilitate heat removal from the patient's body.

■ **100% supplemental oxygen with a nonrebreathing mask**
  - Any patient with an altered mental status must receive 100% supplemental oxygen as soon as possible.
  - Be prepared to provide positive pressure ventilatory assistance if this patient's respirations become shallow.

2. What is your interpretation of this cardiac rhythm?

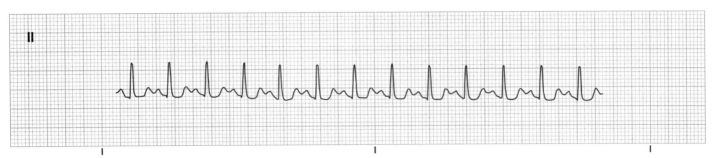

■ **Figure 17-2** Your patient's cardiac rhythm.

This is *sinus tachycardia* **(Figure 17-2)**. The rhythm is regular, has a ventricular rate of 145 beats/min, and monomorphic, upright P waves that consistently precede each narrow QRS complex.

As previously discussed in other case studies within this book, sinus tachycardia is a response to an underlying condition rather than a cardiac dysrhythmia itself. You must therefore carefully and systematically assess the patient, identify the cause, and provide the appropriate treatment.

The patient in this case is tachycardic in response to heat exposure, in which the sympathetic nervous system is responding in an attempt to compensate for the dehydration associated with his heat exposure.

3. What is your field impression of this patient?

This patient is suffering from *exertional heatstroke*. The following assessment findings support this field impression:

■ **Prolonged exposure to heat, for 5 hours.** This, in combination with the high relative humidity, has effectively promoted exertional heatstroke.

■ **Documented hyperthermia of 104.8°F,** which is critically high, and is indicative of uncompensated hyperthermia (hypothalamic failure).

■ **Confusion,** which indicates central nervous system involvement. This is a less common finding in other heat disorders, such as heat exhaustion.

■ **Hot, flushed skin,** which is very characteristic of significant hyperthermia. Although the cessation of sweating is typically seen in patients with heatstroke, perspiration may remain on the skin from previous exertion.

■ **Hypotension and tachycardia,** which reflect significant dehydration.

Before we discuss heatstroke, a brief review of how heat is generated by the body and the mechanisms by which heat is removed from the body is in order.

There are two mechanisms by which the body produces heat — from within the body and from contact with the external environment.

The thermal gradient is the difference between the patient's body temperature and that of the ambient environment. Ambient temperature is generally different (higher or lower) than body temperature. If ambient temperature is higher than body temperature, heat will flow into the body in an attempt to equalize the temperature. Factors such as wind speed and relative humidity also influence heat loss or gain from the body.

Thermogenesis is defined as the generation of heat within the body. Factors that generate heat within the body include physical exercise or exertion, shivering, increased cellular metabolism caused by epinephrine and norepinephrine, and the process of digestion.

In order to maintain stability of the internal environment (homeostasis), the body must be able to release heat to the environment. The process of heat removal from the body is called thermolysis. There are five mechanisms in which body heat is lost to the environment **(Table 17-5)**. Body heat is constantly being lost because the internal body temperature is generally greater than that of the environment.

Table 17-5 Mechanisms for Losing Body Heat

Conduction	Direct contact of the body with another surface
Convection	The loss of heat by air currents passing across the body
Radiation	Removal of heat from the body's surface directly into the environment
Evaporation	Loss of heat as water evaporates from the skin or within the lungs
Respiration	The lungs transfer heat to inhaled air through radiation and convection. Evaporation in the lungs humidifies the air, which is exhaled from the body, thus removing heat.

The mechanisms described in Table 17-5 are utilized by the body to regulate or maintain temperature through a process called thermoregulation, which is regulated by the hypothalamus, located in the brainstem.

Typically, the core body temperature is 98.6° F (37° C); however, the temperature varies from person to person. For example, a person with a rapid metabolic rate would have a higher core body temperature than that of a person with a slow metabolic rate, because the process of metabolism produces heat.

The hypothalamus, as previously mentioned, is the central regulation point for the maintenance of body temperature. Much in the same way that the thermostat in your house operates, the hypothalamus (thermostat) senses changes in body temperature, and, as needed, secretes neurotransmitters that cause the body to produce heat (shivering) or remove heat (sweating) from the body.

Heatstroke occurs when the core body temperature increases and the hypothalamic temperature-regulating mechanism fails. Using the thermostat analogy again—if you turn up (reset) the thermostat in your house to a higher temperature, the air conditioner will not come on until that reset temperature is met. This is essentially what happens to the hypothalamus in heatstroke. As the core body temperature rises, it is reset to a higher "normal" body temperature. Unfortunately, however, heatstroke renders the hypothalamus unable to effectively function; therefore, it cannot activate heat-removing mechanisms. As a result, core body temperature soars, climbing as high as 105° F or higher.

Heatstroke is characterized by severe hyperthermia (105° F or higher) and central nervous system dysfunction. If left untreated, death is almost certain, resulting from damage to the cells and tissues of the brain, kidneys, and liver.

Severe dehydration is also present with heatstroke and is secondary to the depletion of salt and water from the body as it attempts to remove heat through evaporation.

Your patient is experiencing exertional heatstroke, which most often occurs in otherwise healthy people. Prolonged exertion in excessively high ambient temperatures effectively promotes this type of heatstroke. With exertional heatstroke, you will find that although sweating has ceased and the skin is red and hot, residual perspiration may still be present on the patient's body from previous exertion. Do not let this fool you into a field impression of heat exhaustion, which is characterized by cool, moist skin.

Patients with chronic illnesses and older persons often experience what is referred to as classic heatstroke, in which high core body temperatures are uncompensated for because of an age or illness-induced deficiencies in thermoregulatory function. Since exertion is typically not a factor with classic heatstroke, the patient's skin will almost always be hot and dry.

You must perform a rapid, yet systematic assessment of the patient with a heat-related emergency, identify the signs and symptoms of heatstroke **(Table 17-6)**, and provide prompt, aggressive management.

Table 17-6 Signs and Symptoms of Heatstroke

Core body temperature of 105° F or higher
Red, hot skin (dry or moist)
Deep, rapid breathing
Hypotension and tachycardia
Mental status changes ranging from confusion to coma
Seizures in severe cases

4. Are the patient's vital signs and SAMPLE history consistent with your field impression?

The patient's hypotension and tachycardia are consistent with dehydration caused by heatstroke. Additionally, his declining mental status confirms the central nervous system dysfunction that is seen with heatstroke.

The patient's medical history is unremarkable for predisposing factors to classic heatstroke (diabetes, heart disease); however, his prolonged exertion during exposure to high ambient temperatures provides ample information to confirm a field impression of exertional heatstroke.

5. What specific treatment is required for this patient's condition?

Further treatment for this patient is aimed at rapidly lowering his body temperature and replacing lost fluids.

- Rapid, active cooling
  - Remove all clothing; cover the patient with sheets or trauma dressings soaked in tepid water or saline. You can also fan the patient and spray a mist of tepid water over him if you have an atomizer (spray bottle).
    - Monitor the patient's core body temperature during the cooling process.
    - Overcooling the patient may cause him to shiver, which could raise his core body temperature.
    - Ice cold water and chemical icepacks may cause a reflex vasoconstriction that would prevent the patient from releasing body heat, and should thus be avoided.

■ IV fluid replacement
  • Start 2 large-bore (14- to 16-gauge catheters) IV lines.
  • Infuse up to 2 L of normal saline and then reassess the patient.
    ◦ In cases of severe dehydration, up to 3 L of normal saline may be required.

Because of electrolyte derangements, patients with heatstroke are prone to cardiac dysrhythmias; therefore, continuous electrocardiogram monitoring is essential.

Avoid the use of vasopressor drugs (dopamine, norepinephrine) to raise blood pressure because these agents cause vasoconstriction, which may impair sweating.

Continually monitor the patient's airway and breathing and initiate positive pressure ventilatory support if his respirations become shallow.

6. Is further treatment required for this patient?

This patient's condition is clearly improving with your treatment. Continue cooling measures, taking care to avoid overcooling and shivering. Reassess the patient's airway and breathing and make any treatment adjustments as needed. Since the patient's blood pressure has improved, consider setting your IV line(s) to a keep-vein-open rate.

7. Are there any special considerations for this patient?

There is one point regarding heatstroke that deserves special consideration. Although this patient's skin is diaphoretic, his heatstroke is as serious as the person who presents with hot, dry skin. In fact, he is probably not actively sweating, but rather, has residual perspiration from previous exertion. Do not let this finding deter you from making the right field impression.

If patients with a heat-related emergency present like a "Really Hot Cat" (red, hot skin, central nervous system dysfunction), call it heatstroke, whether their skin is moist or not!

Summary

Heatstroke is the deadliest form of heat-related emergency. It occurs when the body produces heat faster than it can be removed, causing the core body temperature to climb to 105° F or higher. You will typically encounter heatstroke when people physically exert themselves for a prolonged period of time in an environment that is hot and humid. Very young people and older people are especially prone to heatstroke because of their decreased ability to activate the appropriate heat-removing mechanisms (eg, sweating, vasodilation). Other factors that predispose a person to heatstroke include hypertension, diabetes, and heart disease.

Treatment involves immediate removal of the patient from the hot environment, managing the airway appropriately, rapidly cooling the body, and replacing lost fluids with normal saline. Prompt transport to the hospital is essential.

You must act quickly when caring for a patient with heatstroke. If the condition is left untreated, death will occur due to vital organ failure.

18

31-Year-Old Male with Bizarre Behavior

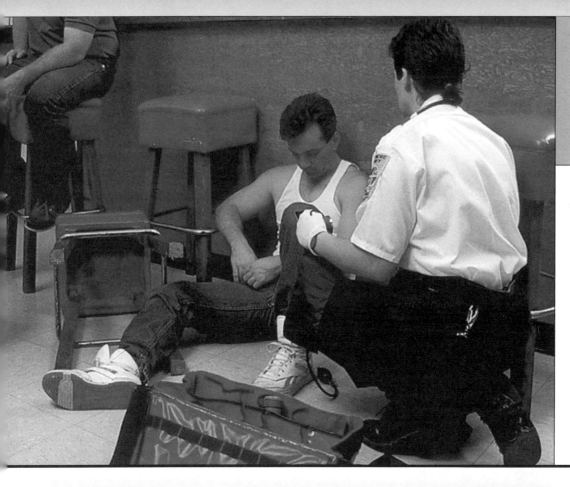

You are dispatched to a local bar at 437 Oak Park St for a 31-year-old male, who, according to the owner of the bar, is "acting strange." The time of call is 10:15 pm. Your response time to the scene is approximately 5 minutes.

You arrive at the scene at 10:20 pm. Law enforcement personnel have already secured the scene. You enter the establishment and find the patient sitting on the floor. He is conscious, though staring at the floor with a blank look. A patron recognizes the patient and tells you that the patient occasionally comes in but never drinks alcohol, just water. You perform an initial assessment **(Table 18-1)** as your partner obtains additional information from the patron.

Table 18-1 Initial Assessment

Level of Consciousness	Conscious, but not talking
Chief Complaint	According to the bar owner, "He walked in and was acting very strange, as though someone were following him. He then sat down on the floor."
Airway and Breathing	Airway, patent; respirations, normal rate and depth
Circulation	Pulse, normal rate, strong and regular; skin, warm and dry

1. What initial management is indicated for this patient?

_____

_____

_____

_____

The patient is offered supplemental oxygen, which he refuses to accept. Although his speech pattern is disorganized, it is not slurred. He tells you that a black car has been following him for the last week. There are no strange odors noted on the patient's breath.

The patient has his fist against his chest. You ask him if his chest hurts, but he does not answer you. You perform a focused history and physical examination **(Table 18-2)** on the patient. He is disinterested in what you are doing, but he cooperates.

Table 18-2 Focused History and Physical Examination

Description of the Episode	According to the bar owner, "acting strange"
Onset	Unknown
Duration	Unknown
Associated Symptoms	Possible chest pain, bizarre behavior, disorganized speech pattern
Evidence of Trauma	None
Interventions Prior to EMS Arrival	None
Seizures	No seizures were witnessed by the patron or bar owner.
Blood Glucose	101 mg/dL
Oxygen Saturation	99% (on room air)
Fever	The patient is afebrile.

With the patient's permission, you attach the ECG leads and obtain a cardiac rhythm strip **(Figure 18-1)**. Again, you ask him if he is having chest pain, but he still will not answer you. He asks your partner to go outside to "see if the black car is there."

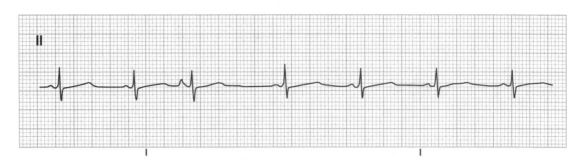

■ **Figure 18-1** Your patient's cardiac rhythm.

2. What is your interpretation of this cardiac rhythm?

_____

_____

_____

The patient continues to remain calm throughout your assessment. He allows you to obtain baseline vital signs and perform a SAMPLE history **(Table 18-3)**.

Table 18-3 Baseline Vital Signs and SAMPLE History

Blood Pressure	128/66 mm Hg
Pulse	74 beats/min, strong and occasionally irregular
Respirations	16 breaths/min and unlabored
Oxygen Saturation	99% (on room air)
Signs and Symptoms	Disorganized speech, paranoid behavior
Allergies	"No, I'm not allergic to any drugs."
Medications	Zyprexa
Pertinent Past History	"The doctor thinks that I am crazy, and that I should see him every month. I think that he just wants my money. I'm not sick, and never have been."
Last Oral Intake	"I'm not hungry. I can't remember when I last ate."
Events Leading to Present Illness	"That black car followed me here. I came inside to hide from it."

3. What is your field impression of this patient?

_____

_____

_____

_____

4. Are the patient's vital signs and SAMPLE history consistent with your field impression?

_____

_____

_____

You advise the patient of the need to be transported to the emergency department for evaluation. He refuses to allow you to take him anywhere, and accuses you of wanting to take him to the "funny farm."

5. What specific treatment is required for this patient's condition?

_____

_____

_____

Following repeated assurances that you are concerned about his physical well-being and that you will transport him to the emergency department, the patient eventually agrees to transport. On his own accord, he walks to the ambulance. The police officer discreetly follows you to the hospital in the event that the patient turns violent. En route, you perform an ongoing assessment **(Table 18-4)** and then call your radio report to the receiving hospital.

Table 18-4 Ongoing Assessment	
Level of Consciousness	Conscious, but minimally talkative
Airway and Breathing	Respirations, 16 breaths/min and unlabored
Oxygen Saturation	99% (on room air)
Blood Pressure	130/70 mm Hg
Pulse	78 beats/min, strong and occasionally irregular
Mood and Affect	Minimally talkative, calm

6. Is further treatment required for this patient?

_____

_____

_____

_____

7. Are there any special considerations for this patient?

_____

_____

_____

The patient is delivered to the emergency department without incident. You give your verbal report to the attending physician.

After ruling out physical causes of his condition, the patient is evaluated in the emergency department by a resident psychiatrist. The patient admits he has not been compliant with his medication. Following additional assessment, he is admitted to the psychiatric unit for stabilization of his crisis.

1. What initial management is indicated for this patient?

- **Paramedic safety**
  - When managing a potential psychiatric emergency, you must realize that the situation can quickly turn violent. Therefore, maintaining a safe distance from the patient and being prepared for a quick retreat are extremely important.

- **Patience**
  - It is clear that this patient is going to require some time to answer your questions. Being patient will often help you obtain the information you need. Do not, however, force the issue if the patient absolutely refuses to answer specific questions.

- **Supplemental oxygen**
  - Although it appears that this patient is experiencing a psychiatric crisis, his disorganized speech pattern should be assumed to be the result of hypoxia until proven otherwise.
  - *Offer* the patient supplemental oxygen, either with a nonrebreathing mask or nasal cannula, but certainly do not force any therapy if the patient refuses.

2. What is your interpretation of this cardiac rhythm?

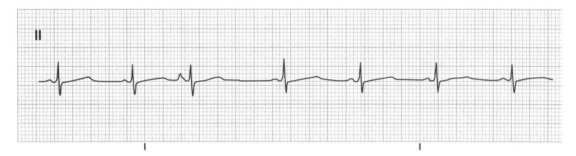

■ **Figure 18-2** Your patient's cardiac rhythm.

The underlying rhythm, a sinus rhythm, is characterized by a regular rhythm, a ventricular rate of approximately 75 beats/min, and upright, monomorphic P waves that consistently precede each narrow QRS complex **(Figure 18-2)**. There is, however, a premature complex (third complex from the left). Because of the narrow QRS complex, the rhythm is supraventricular in origin. The P wave, although upright, takes on a different morphology from the P waves in the rest of the rhythm. This rhythm should therefore be interpreted as a *sinus rhythm with one premature atrial complex (PAC)*.

A PAC occurs when an ectopic focus in the atrium generates an impulse in the midst of an otherwise normal rhythm. Because the impulse does not originate in the sinoatrial node, the P wave that precedes it will look differently than other, normally conducted complexes. Because the PAC occurs "out of line," so to speak, it will be obviously premature, breaking the cadence of the underlying rhythm.

PACs are commonly the result of excessive caffeine and/or nicotine intake. They rarely cause hemodynamic compromise in a patient, who is usually unaware of their presence. PACs also occur in perfectly healthy individuals, even in the absence of caffeine or nicotine intake.

Numerous PACs could, however, indicate a more serious problem in the atria. If frequent enough, they could precipitate a supraventricular tachycardia (SVT).

In the case of this patient, there does not appear to be a correlation between this benign cardiac rhythm and his present condition.

3. What is your field impression of this patient?

This patient's behavior is consistent with *schizophrenia*. The following assessment findings support this field impression:

- **Blank stare and disinterested attitude**, which is referred to as a flat affect, and is frequently seen in schizophrenic patients.

- **Disorganized speech pattern**, which, in schizophrenic patients, can also be accompanied by disorganized behavior or appearance (eg, the way they dress).

- **Apparent paranoia**, as evidenced by his concerns that a black car has been following him.

Schizophrenia is a common psychiatric disorder characterized by recurrent alterations in behavior, including delusions, hallucinations, and depression. The schizophrenic patient has lost contact with reality and is preoccupied with his or her own inner fantasies. Although several theories exist, the definitive cause of schizophrenia is unknown.

Approximately 2 million adult Americans have been diagnosed with schizophrenia, which affects both sexes equally. The disorder typically presents in males in their late teens to early 20s and females in their late 20s to early 30s. Unfortunately, 1 of 10 patients diagnosed with schizophrenia will eventually commit suicide.

According to the *Diagnostic and Statistical Manual of Psychiatric Disorders*, 4th Edition text revised (*DSM-IV-TR*), published by the American Psychiatric Association, a diagnosis of schizophrenia is made if a patient exhibits two or more Criterion A symptoms **(Table 18-5)**, which are present for a significant portion of time during a 1-month period (less if successfully treated).

Table 18-5 Criterion A Symptoms of Schizophrenia

Delusions
- Fixed, false beliefs that are out of context based on the patient's religious or cultural group.

Hallucinations
- Sensory perceptions with no realistic basis (eg, hearing voices, seeing things)

Disorganized (derailed) speech or incoherence

Grossly disorganized, bizarre, or catatonic behavior

Negative symptoms
- Flat affect: Disinterested appearance, lack of facial expression
- Alogia: Limited speech or speech that exceeds the thought content it conveys
- Avolition: Lack of initiative or motivation in achieving a goal

Note: Only one Criterion A symptom is required if delusions are bizarre or hallucinations consist of a voice that maintains a running commentary on the person's behavior or thoughts, or two or more voices conversing with each other.

The *DSM-IV-TR* further categorizes schizophrenia into five subtypes **(Table 18-6)**, each of which has its own diagnostic criteria. Some patients may initially be seen with symptoms from more than one subtype.

Table 18-6 Subtypes of Schizophrenia

Paranoid type
- Preoccupation with one or more delusions or frequent auditory hallucinations
- None of the following is prominent: Disorganized speech, disorganized or catatonic behavior, or flat or inappropriate affect

Catatonic type
- A type of schizophrenia characterized by at least two of the following:
  - Catalepsy: A state of suspended animation and loss of voluntary motion
  - Negativism or mutism
  - Inappropriate or bizarre posture
  - Echolalia: Repetition of what is said by other people as if echoing them
  - Echopraxia: Imitative repetition of the movements, gestures, or posture of others

Disorganized type
- All of the following are prominent:
  - Disorganized speech
  - Disorganized behavior
  - Flat or inappropriate affect
- The criteria are *not* met for the catatonic type.

Undifferentiated type
- A type of schizophrenia in which Criterion A symptoms are present, but the criteria are *not met* for the paranoid, disorganized, or catatonic type.

Residual type
- Absence of prominent delusions, hallucinations, disorganized speech, and grossly disorganized or catatonic behavior
- There is continuing evidence of the disturbance, as indicated by the presence of negative symptoms, or two or more symptoms listed in Criterion A for schizophrenia that are present in an attenuated form (odd beliefs, unusual perceptual experiences).

Many patients with schizophrenia, as well as those with other psychiatric disorders, live relatively normal lives, providing they are compliant with their prescribed medications.

Like many other disease processes (physical and psychological), medication noncompliance is perhaps the most common cause of the acute psychotic episodes associated with schizophrenia.

4. Are the patient's vital signs and SAMPLE history consistent with your field impression?

This patient's vital signs are within normal limits and are thus not relevant to his current condition. His medical history, on the other hand, tells a different story.

The statement that the "doctor thinks I'm crazy" indicates a distorted perception of the physician's actual diagnosis. The statement that "I think he just wants my money" reinforces this patient's paranoid behavior. The fact that the patient is seen (or at least should be seen) on a monthly basis indicates that his schizophrenia is not as controlled as it should be. As previously mentioned, provided that schizophrenic patients comply with their medication regimens, they typically live relatively normal lives.

Finally, the patient's medication is used to treat not only schizophrenia, but a number of other psychiatric disorders as well.

- **Olanzapine (Zyprexa)** is an antipsychotic agent that belongs to the thienobenzodiazepine class of drugs. It is used to treat a variety of psychiatric disorders, including schizophrenia and bipolar disorder. Although the exact mechanism of action of Zyprexa is unknown, it is believed to antagonize dopamine and serotonin receptors in the brain, both of which play key roles in a patient's mood and affect.

Other medications used in the treatment of schizophrenia include haloperidol (Haldol), risperidone (Risperdal), clozapine (Clozaril), and quetiapine (Seroquel).

5. What specific treatment is required for this patient's condition?

First and foremost, you must ensure continued safety of yourself and your partner, as paranoid reactions can quickly lead to violent behavior. General guidelines, which will maximize your safety, include:

- **Ensure the presence of law enforcement**, both before and during your presence at the scene.
- **Maintain a position that is between the patient and an exit.** Never allow the patient to block your potential escape route. If the situation turns violent, you will be unable to make a hasty retreat.
- **Plan your escape route before you need it.** The front door may seem to be the most obvious escape route, but it may not be the closest. Look for alternate exits from the building.

Signs that the patient may become violent include, but are not limited to, an increase in the volume and quickness of speech, clenching fists, and a threatening stance. Remain alert for these signs of potential violence.

General management of patients with schizophrenia includes the following:

- **Clearly identify yourself as a paramedic.** Many paranoid schizophrenics may think that you are a police officer and that you are going to take them to jail.
- **Be friendly, yet distant and neutral** while expressing your intent to help the patient. Do not be overly friendly, as patients may interpret this as an attempt to gain their confidence for ulterior motives.
- **Avoid furthering the patient's paranoia** by actions such as speaking with family members or bystanders in a hushed or secretive tone.
- **Do not play along with hallucinations**, as this will only serve to reinforce the patient's unrealistic perceptions.
- **Do not respond to the patient's anger**, unless it presents an immediate threat to your safety and self-defense is necessary.
- **Be tactful and firm** as you persuade the patient to allow you to transport him or her to the hospital.

If the patient is uncooperative or violent, physical restraint may be necessary. If restraint is needed, law enforcement needs to get involved. Medical control may request that you administer an antipsychotic agent (eg, Haldol). Refer to locally established protocols regarding pharmacological treatment of psychiatric disorders in the field. Your first priority, should the patient turn violent, is to ensure your own safety.

6. Is further treatment required for this patient?

Continue to talk with the patient, but do not fear silence if the patient elects not to speak to you. Forcing a psychiatric patient to talk may only lead to agitation and an increased potential for violent behavior.

7. Are there any special considerations for this patient?

If this patient becomes uncooperative or violent while en route to the hospital, you must instruct your partner to stop the ambulance immediately. The police officer who is following you may have to accompany you in the back of the ambulance, and physical or pharmacological restraint may be needed. Physical restraint of a patient should generally not be attempted unless you have sufficient personnel (one person per extremity); therefore, additional help would be required should physical restraint become necessary.

Keeping your guard up and remaining aware of the patient's actions cannot be overemphasized. Although the patient is calm at present, this could change without warning.

Summary

Schizophrenia is a common psychiatric disorder, affecting an estimated 2 million adult Americans. Although not fully understood in terms of its etiology, schizophrenia is characterized by recurrent episodes of psychotic behavior, which may include delusions, hallucinations, and paranoid behavior.

Patients with schizophrenia often have a family history of the disorder. If affects both males and females equally, and most commonly presents in early adulthood.

Patients with schizophrenia may lead relatively normal lives unless they are noncompliant with their medications (Zyprexa, Haldol). However, breakthrough episodes of abnormal behavior can occur despite medication compliance.

Management for the patient with a schizophrenic episode begins by ensuring the safety of yourself and your partner. Law enforcement presence is important in the event that the patient suddenly turns violent.

Maintain a professional and nonjudgmental attitude with the patient, and avoid actions that may further paranoid behavior or reinforce auditory or visual hallucinations.

If the patient becomes violent, physical restraint and/or pharmacological intervention may be necessary. In general, restraint of a patient should not be attempted unless there are adequate personnel available (one person per extremity). Call for additional help if physical restraint becomes necessary.

19

65-Year-Old Male with Chest Pain and Dyspnea

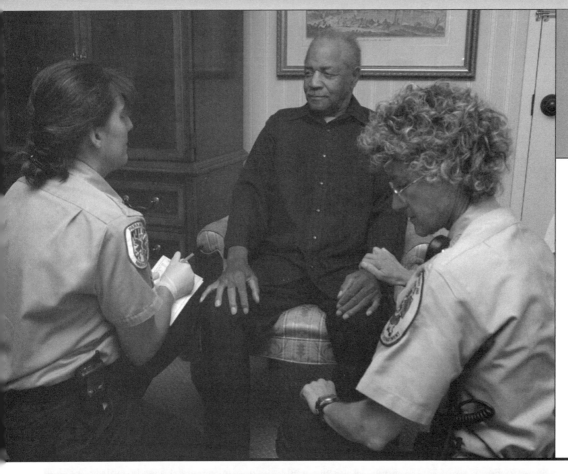

At 9:33 am, your unit is dispatched to a private residence at 518 West Turner St for a 65-year-old male who is complaining of chest pain and shortness of breath. Your response time to the scene is less than 2 minutes.

You arrive at the scene at 9:35 am, and enter the patient's residence. You find him sitting in a chair in his living room. He appears anxious, is mildly dyspneic, and tells you that he has a sharp pain in his chest. You perform an initial assessment **(Table 19-1)** as your partner obtains additional information from his wife.

Table 19-1 Initial Assessment

Level of Consciousness	Conscious and alert to person, place, and time, anxious
Chief Complaint	"I have a sharp pain in the left side of my chest, and it is a little hard to breathe."
Airway and Breathing	Airway, patent; respirations, increased and mildly labored; adequate tidal volume
Circulation	Pulse, strong, occasionally irregular, normal rate; skin, warm and dry

1. What initial management is indicated for this patient?

_____

_____

_____

_____

After completing the initial management for this patient, you perform a focused history and physical examination **(Table 19-2)**. The patient remains conscious and alert and is able to provide you with the required information. Your partner proceeds to attach the ECG leads to the patient's chest.

Table 19-2 Focused History and Physical Examination

Onset	"This started suddenly."
Provocation/Palliation	"The pain gets worse when I take a deep breath."
Quality	"It is very sharp, like someone is sticking a knife in my chest."
Radiation/Referred Pain	"The pain stays in the left side of my chest and does not move anywhere else. I also have pain in my left calf."
Severity	"It hurts badly when I take in a deep breath."
Time	"This started about 30 minutes ago."
Interventions Prior to EMS Arrival	"I thought that maybe I had slept wrong, so I placed a heating pad on my chest. It did not help."
Chest Exam	Chest wall moves symmetrically, no retractions are noted.
Breath Sounds	Equal bilaterally, isolated wheezing is heard over the left lower lobe of the lung
Jugular Veins	Normal
Oxygen Saturation	98% (on 100% oxygen)
Temperature	100.4° F

Your partner runs a 6-second strip of the patient's cardiac rhythm **(Figure 19-1)** and hands it to you for evaluation. The patient tells you that he would like for you to take him to the hospital, so your partner retrieves the stretcher from the ambulance.

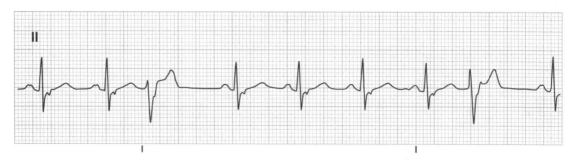

■ **Figure 19-1** Your patient's cardiac rhythm.

2. What is your interpretation of this cardiac rhythm?

_____

_____

_____

_____

An IV line of normal saline is established and set at a keep-vein-open rate. After placing the patient in a full Fowler's position on the stretcher, you obtain baseline vital signs and a SAMPLE history **(Table 19-3)**. The patient remains conscious, alert, and mildly dyspneic.

Table 19-3 Baseline Vital Signs and SAMPLE History

Blood Pressure	148/88 mm Hg
Pulse	88 beats/min, strong, occasionally irregular
Respirations	22 breaths/min, mildly labored, adequate tidal volume
Oxygen Saturation	98% (on 100% oxygen)
Signs and Symptoms	Sharp chest pain worsened with inhalation, pain in the left calf muscle.
Allergies	"I am allergic to ibuprofen and penicillin."
Medications	"I take vitamins and Coreg."
Pertinent Past History	"I had my left hip replaced 2 years ago. I also have high blood pressure."
Last Oral Intake	"I had a bowl of cereal 2 or 3 hours ago."
Events Leading to Present Illness	"My left calf had been hurting for the last 2 or 3 days."

The patient further tells you that since his hip replacement, he has been less able to ambulate, and is not as active as he was before.

3. What is your field impression of this patient?

_____

_____

_____

_____

4. Are the patient's vital signs and SAMPLE history consistent with your field impression?

_____

_____

_____

_____

The patient is loaded into the ambulance, and transport to the hospital is begun. Further treatment and monitoring are continued en route. Your estimated time of arrival at the receiving hospital is approximately 15 minutes.

5. What specific treatment is required for this patient's condition?

_____

_____

_____

_____

The patient remains conscious and alert and in mild respiratory distress. However, he is not as restless since you began the oxygen therapy. You perform an ongoing assessment **(Table 19-4)** and then call your radio report to the receiving hospital.

Table 19-4 Ongoing Assessment

Level of Consciousness	Conscious and alert to person, place, and time
Airway and Breathing	Respirations, 22 breaths/min, mildly labored; adequate tidal volume
Oxygen Saturation	98% (on 100% oxygen)
Blood Pressure	150/88 mm Hg
Pulse	90 beats/min, strong and occasionally irregular
Breath Sounds	Bilaterally equal, isolated wheezing to the left lower lobe of the lung
Jugular Veins	Normal

6. Is further treatment required for this patient?

_____

_____

_____

_____

7. Are there any special considerations for this patient?

_____

_____

_____

_____

_____

Delivery of the patient to the emergency department staff occurs without incident. You give your verbal report to the charge nurse.

Arterial blood gas analysis reveals a slightly low level of arterial partial pressure of oxygen, and a ventilation-quantification (VQ) scan reveals a small pulmonary embolism in the lower lobe of his left lung. Further assessment yields a diagnosis of a left lower extremity deep venous thrombosis. An infusion of heparin is initiated and the patient is admitted to the medical intensive care unit.

A TED hose is applied to help control swelling in the leg and he is placed on oral coumadin. After an uneventful 5-day stay in the hospital, the patient is discharged home.

CASE STUDY ANSWERS AND SUMMARY

1. What initial management is indicated for this patient?

- 100% supplemental oxygen with a nonrebreathing mask
  - Any patient with chest pain and/or dyspnea should receive 100% supplemental oxygen as soon as possible.
  - Although much less common, an acute coronary syndrome can present with pain is described as being sharp. Atypical chest pain is common in older persons, who may perceive pain differently than younger adults.

2. What is your interpretation of this cardiac rhythm?

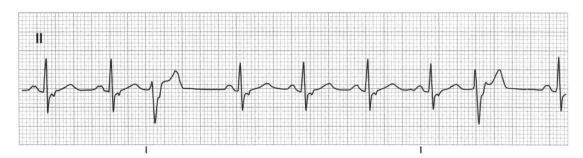

■ **Figure 19-2** Your patient's cardiac rhythm.

The underlying rhythm is sinus, as evidenced by the presence of monomorphic P waves that are consistently followed by narrow QRS complexes **(Figure 19-2)**. The ventricular rate is approximately 85 beats/min. There are, however, two premature complexes, neither of which has preceding P waves. The premature complexes both start with positive waves that are identical to the start of the sinus QRS complexes, indicating that they are junctional in origin. Then, aberrancy (abnormal conduction) develops, as evidenced by the acute widening of the premature complexes. This would account for their different QRS morphologies. This rhythm is interpreted as a sinus rhythm with two *premature junctional complexes (PJCs)*.

A PJC is caused by an ectopic focus within the AV junction. In the context of a sinus rhythm, a PJC will appear as an obviously premature complex, thus breaking the cadence of the underlying rhythm. P waves may or may not be present. If present, P waves will be inverted because of retrograde conduction into the atrium. P waves may also be seen after the QRS complex.

P waves that precede the QRS complex most likely originate in the proximal portion of the AV junction. P waves that occur during or after the QRS complex most likely originate in the distal portion of the AV junction.

Isolated PJCs may occur idiopathically in healthy people. They could, however, indicate AV nodal disease, hypoxia, or acute myocardial infarction (among others).

Frequent PJCs (> 6 per minute) may indicate a reentry mechanism in the AV junction, which could lead to a more serious junctional dysrhythmia (eg, junctional tachycardia).

In the case of this patient, there does not appear to be a correlation between the PJCs and his present condition.

3. What is your field impression of this patient?

This patient is experiencing an acute *pulmonary embolism (PE)*. The following assessment findings support this field impression:

- **Sudden onset of pleuritic chest pain**, which is extremely common in patients with an acute PE.

- **Dyspnea**, which is secondary to decreased air movement in the portion of the lung that is not being perfused.

- **Localized wheezing**, which indicates bronchoconstriction localized to the area of the embolism.

- **Calf pain**, which is caused by a deep venous thrombosis (DVT), from where the thrombus likely detached.

An acute pulmonary embolism refers to the blockage of one or more pulmonary arteries by a blood clot (thrombus) or other foreign material that breaks free from a distant location and travels to the heart. The most common origin of the thrombus is a large vein in the lower extremity, where a DVT or blood stagnation has occurred. Other causes of acute PE include air, fatty tissue, and amniotic fluid.

The embolism, upon returning to the right side of the heart, enters the pulmonary vasculature and lodges in a pulmonary artery **(Figure 19-3)**. If the pulmonary artery is partially obstructed, lung tissue distal to the obstruction becomes ischemic. Necrosis of the distal lung tissue occurs if the pulmonary artery is completely obstructed.

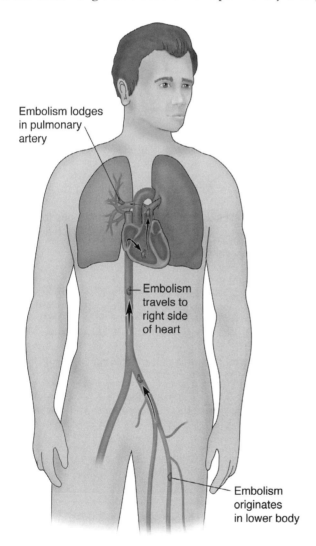

Embolism lodges in pulmonary artery

Embolism travels to right side of heart

Embolism originates in lower body

■ **Figure 19-3** Pulmonary embolism from a lower extremity thrombus.

The signs and symptoms of an acute PE depend on both the size of the embolus and the pulmonary artery that it obstructs.

Small pulmonary emboli typically present with acute mild dyspnea, pleuritic (sharp) chest pain localized over the area of affected lung tissue that increases with deep inhalation, and restlessness that reflects mild to moderate hypoxia. Some patients with small emboli may not present with dyspnea, only pleuritic chest pain.

Because the lung area distal to the pulmonary arterial blockage is being ventilated but not perfused (ventilation-perfusion mismatch), a reflex bronchoconstriction secondary to local hypocarbia may occur. For this reason, some patients with an acute PE may be initially seen with wheezing that is auscultated over the area of the affected lung tissue.

Large emboli typically present with more severe acute dyspnea and pleuritic chest pain. However, since a larger pulmonary artery has been obstructed, pulmonary hypertension and acute right-sided heart failure (cor pulmonale) often result. Jugular venous distention therefore may be present. Significant hypoxia and hypercarbia cause cyanosis, hypotension, and tachycardia, and sometimes cause the patient to become unconscious.

A massive PE often results in sudden death secondary to a complete or near-complete cessation of oxygenation. The presentation typically includes a sudden onset of profound labored breathing, upper torso cyanosis, and cardiopulmonary arrest.

There are numerous risk factors for a PE **(Table 19-5)** that require the paramedic to perform a careful, systematic patient assessment. Many patients with pulmonary emboli are misdiagnosed, even in the hospital setting.

Table 19-5 Risk Factors for Pulmonary Embolism

Limited mobility
- Patients who live a sedentary lifestyle or were recently hospitalized with prolonged bed rest
  - Blood stagnates in the lower extremities, which increases the risk of thrombus formation.
  - These patients are especially prone to a deep venous thrombosis, from which a clot may dislodge.

Thrombophlebitis
- Venous inflammation accompanied by a thrombus

Atrial fibrillation
- Blood in the fibrillating atria can stagnate and form microemboli, which are ejected from the right ventricle and lodge in a pulmonary artery.

Recent surgery
- Pulmonary emboli often result from fatty tissue that breaks free from the surgical site following hip or lower extremity surgery.

Long bone fractures
- Fatty tissue can be released from the bone marrow of the fractured bone and travels as an embolism.

Use of oral contraceptives
- Oral contraceptives have been linked to hypercoagulability, which increases the patient's risk of developing a PE. Contraception use in conjunction with cigarette smoking places the patient in an even higher risk category.

Pregnancy
- Although a less common cause of acute PE, amniotic fluid can enter the maternal circulation during or after delivery. Amniotic fluid emboli are often fatal.

Blood disorders
- Polycythemia vera is a rare blood disorder characterized by an increased number of red blood cells, which increases the likelihood of blood clotting.

Because you suspect that this patient's PE is secondary to a DVT, the patient should be evaluated for Homan's sign. Homan's sign is characterized by increased pain in the calf muscle upon dorsiflexion of the foot, and is a hallmark finding of a DVT. The affected leg may be edematous as well because of decreased venous return.

4. Are the patient's vital signs and SAMPLE history consistent with your field impression?

This patient's vital signs are remarkable for low-grade fever which is present in a majority of patients with acute PE. Although his respirations are somewhat labored and increased, which is typical of an acute PE, his heart rate is not tachycardic as one might expect it to be. This is likely the result of his alpha-beta-blocking antihypertensive medication, which, by suppressing the sympathetic nervous system, is preventing the typical tachycardia commonly associated with acute PE.

- **Carvedilol** (Coreg) is an alpha- and beta-adrenergic antagonist used to treat hypertension. Lowering of the blood pressure is secondary to decreased myocardial contractility, vasodilation, and, after approximately 4 weeks of treatment, decreased plasma levels of renin, a potent vasoconstrictor.

The patient's recent history of calf muscle pain is a hallmark finding of a DVT, which is where the embolism likely originated. Patients who are less mobile (elderly, post-surgical patients) are especially prone to the development of a lower extremity thrombus secondary to blood stagnation. Findings suggestive of a DVT (calf pain, Homan's sign) are present in up to 50% of patients with acute PE.

5. What specific treatment is required for this patient's condition?

Although this patient's symptomatology does not suggest a large pulmonary embolism, another thrombus could easily detach from his lower extremity, obstruct a larger pulmonary artery, and quickly cause his condition to deteriorate. Treatment at this point is the same as for any patient with an acute respiratory emergency:

- **Continue 100% oxygen therapy**, which will prevent or treat hypoxemia.
- **Monitor for signs of inadequate breathing (severely labored, shallow depth)**, and be prepared to assist ventilations if necessary. If the patient becomes unconscious, endotracheal intubation may be necessary.
- **Monitor the ECG** for hypoxia-induced cardiac dysrhythmias and be prepared to initiate CPR if cardiac arrest occurs.

6. Is further treatment required for this patient?

As evidenced by the decrease in his restlessness, the oxygen therapy appears to be successfully addressing this patient's hypoxia. At this point, no further treatment interventions are required. Continually monitor his airway status, vital signs, and ECG, and be prepared to adjust treatment accordingly.

7. Are there any special considerations for this patient?

This patient is a potential candidate for fibrinolytic therapy. The Food and Drug Administration has currently approved three fibrinolytic agents for use with acute PE—streptokinase (Streptase), recombinant tissue plasminogen activator (rtPA), and urokinase (Abbokinase). The goals of treating an acute PE with fibrinolytic agents include early lysis (destruction) of the clot with quicker reperfusion of lung tissue and the prevention of recurring emboli by eliminating the source of the thrombus (DVT).

Fibrinolytic agents, if used in the treatment of acute PE, are commonly administered in conjunction with anticoagulant therapy, such as heparin.

The exclusion criteria (contraindications) for fibrinolytic therapy can be reviewed by referring to the summary in Case Study 1 (page 10).

Summary

Acute PE is a relatively common disorder that affects approximately 600,000 to 700,000 Americans a year. Roughly 10% of patients with acute PE will die, generally within the first hour following obstruction of the pulmonary artery.

Acute PE frequently originates from a DVT in a lower extremity. The thrombus breaks free from the lower extremity and travels to the pulmonary vasculature. Although less common, air, fatty tissue, and amniotic fluid in the pulmonary artery can result in acute PE.

You should suspect an acute PE in patients initially seen with acute dyspnea and pleuritic chest pain. Index of suspicion should increase even further if the patient has a history of pulmonary emboli or predisposing conditions such as a DVT or prolonged immobilization.

Massive pulmonary emboli are frequently associated with cardiac arrest and may result in pulseless electrical activity (PEA), a condition in which a cardiac rhythm presents on the ECG monitor, but the patient does not have a palpable pulse.

Management goals for a patient with an acute PE focus on ensuring a patent airway, administering 100% supplemental oxygen or positive pressure ventilatory assistance if needed, IV therapy, ECG monitoring, and rapid transport to the emergency department. Certain fibrinolytic agents may be of potential benefit to the patient, provided they meet the inclusion criteria.

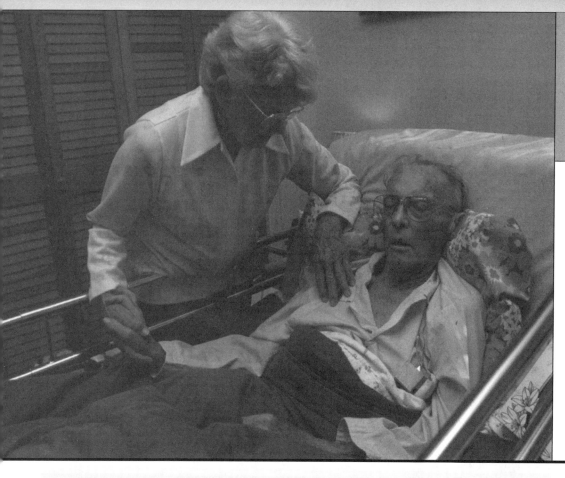

20

72-Year-Old Male with Mental Status Changes

At 3:50 pm, you are dispatched to a nursing care facility at 711 E Schweppe St for a 72-year-old male, who, according to the nursing staff, has "mental status changes." Your response time to the scene is approximately 6 minutes.

Upon arriving at the scene, you enter the patient's room and find him accompanied by his wife. The patient is semiconscious and his respirations appear to be rapid and shallow. As you perform an initial assessment **(Table 20-1)**, the nurse brings you the patient's medical records.

Table 20-1 Initial Assessment

Level of Consciousness	Responsive to painful stimuli only
Chief Complaint	According to the charge nurse, "His mental status has changed over the last 8 hours. He is normally very talkative and alert."
Airway and Breathing	Airway, patent; respirations, rapid and shallow
Circulation	Radial pulse, rate appears normal but is weak and irregular; skin, warm and dry with poor turgor

1. What initial management is indicated for this patient?

_____

_____

_____

_____

Your partner initiates the appropriate management for the patient. With the assistance of the charge nurse and information in the patient's medical records, you perform a focused history and physical examination **(Table 20-2)**. A police officer arrives at the scene to see if you need assistance. You ask him to retrieve the stretcher from the ambulance. The nurse tells you that the patient had a scheduled appointment the next day with his endocrinologist for routine lab work, in follow-up for Addison's disease.

Table 20-2 Focused History and Physical Examination

Description of Episode	"His level of consciousness has progressively declined over the last 8 hours."
Onset	"This has progressed slowly, over the last 8 hours."
Duration	"This was first noticed when he awoke, approximately 8 hours ago."
Associated Symptoms	"He had several episodes of vomiting and diarrhea yesterday afternoon. He was also running a low-grade fever, for which we gave him Motrin."
Evidence of Trauma	None
Interventions Prior to EMS Arrival	"We called his physician, who told us to call EMS immediately."
Seizures	"He has not had any seizures."
Temperature	101.5° F
Oxygen Saturation	97% (ventilated with 100% oxygen)
Blood Glucose	38 mg/dL
Pupils	Equal and sluggishly reactive to light

Your partner continues appropriate management of the patient's airway. You attach the ECG leads to the patient's chest and obtain a 6-second tracing of his cardiac rhythm **(Figure 20-1)**.

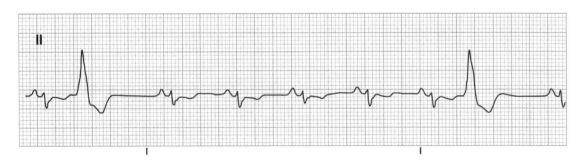

■ **Figure 20-1** Your patient's cardiac rhythm.

2. What is your interpretation of this cardiac rhythm?

_____

_____

_____

_____

After initiating an IV line of normal saline, you administer 25 g of 50% dextrose to treat the patient's hypoglycemia. His mental status has improved somewhat following the dextrose; however, he remains disoriented. A repeat check of his blood glucose reveals a reading of 56 mg/dL. You quickly obtain baseline vital signs and a SAMPLE history **(Table 20-3)**.

Table 20-3 Baseline Vital Signs and SAMPLE History

Blood Pressure	60/40 mm Hg
Pulse	80 beats/min, weak and irregular
Respirations	28 breaths/min and shallow (baseline), although he is being ventilated at 15 breaths/min by your partner
Oxygen Saturation	98% (ventilated with 100% oxygen)
Signs and Symptoms	Altered mental status, hypoglycemia, fever, diarrhea, vomiting, weakness
Allergies	Tetracycline and aspirin
Medications	Cortef and Florinef
Pertinent Past History	Addison's disease
Last Oral Intake	According to the nurse, "He has not eaten anything in the last 24 hours. He told us that he was not hungry."
Events Leading to Present Illness	Vomiting, diarrhea, weakness, and fever since yesterday

3. What is your field impression of this patient?

_____

_____

_____

_____

4. Are the patient's vital signs and SAMPLE history consistent with your field impression?

_____

_____

_____

_____

The patient is placed onto the ambulance stretcher, loaded into the ambulance, and transported immediately. You elect to perform additional interventions en route to the hospital.

5. What specific treatment is required for this patient's condition?

_____

_____

_____

_____

Following additional therapy en route to the hospital, the patient's mental status has improved, and he will no longer tolerate positive pressure ventilations. A nonrebreathing mask is applied and set at 15 L/min. A repeat blood glucose level reveals a reading of 88 mg/dL. You perform an ongoing assessment **(Table 20-4)**, followed by a radio report to the receiving facility.

Table 20-4 Ongoing Assessment

Level of Consciousness	Conscious, still slightly disoriented
Airway and Breathing	Respirations, 20 breaths/min; adequate tidal volume
Oxygen Saturation	98% (on 100% oxygen)
Blood Pressure	100/58 mm Hg
Pulse	84 beats/min, slightly weak but regular
ECG	Normal sinus rhythm
Blood Glucose	88 mg/dL
Pupils	Equal and reactive to light

6. Is further treatment required for this patient?

_____

_____

_____

_____

7. Are there any special considerations for this patient?

_____

_____

_____

_____

The patient is delivered to the emergency department without incident. You give your verbal report to the attending physician. After further assessment, the patient is administered corticosteroids IV and admitted to the medical intensive care unit.

Following a 10-day stay in the hospital for electrolyte stabilization, fluid rehydration, and further corticosteroid treatment, he is discharged back to the nursing care facility.

CASE STUDY ANSWERS AND SUMMARY

1. What initial management is indicated for this patient?

- **Positive pressure ventilations (bag-valve-mask device or pocket mask device)**
  - Rapid, shallow (reduced tidal volume) respirations in conjunction with an altered mental status clearly indicate inadequate breathing and the need for positive pressure ventilatory support.
  - A nasopharyngeal airway should be inserted to assist in maintaining airway patency.
  - Preparations for endotracheal intubation should be made because this patient is at risk for aspiration.

2. What is your interpretation of this cardiac rhythm?

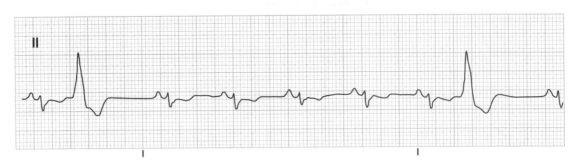

- **Figure 20-2** Your patient's cardiac rhythm.

The underlying rhythm is sinus in origin, as evidenced by the underlying regularity of the rhythm, a ventricular rate of approximately 80 beats/min, and monomorphic P waves that are upright and consistently precede each QRS complex **(Figure 20-2)**. The QRS complexes of the sinus complexes are somewhat wide. This likely indicates an intraventricular conduction delay (eg, bundle branch block).

There are, however, two premature complexes in this rhythm. The premature complexes are wide and bizarre, and are of the same morphology. This rhythm is interpreted as a *sinus rhythm with uniformed premature ventricular complexes (PVCs)*.

A PVC originates from an ectopic pacemaker within the ventricles. As with any electrical impulse that is ventricular in origin, the QRS complex will appear wide (> 0.12 seconds) and have a bizarre appearance. The complex will be obviously premature, occurring earlier than the next expected complex of the underlying rhythm.

PVCs that all have the same morphology are referred to as uniformed PVCs, indicating that they have most likely originated from or near the same ectopic ventricular pacemaker. PVCs of varying morphologies (multiformed) are indicative of more than one ventricular ectopic pacemaker.

Occasional PVCs may occur in healthy people with apparently healthy hearts and without apparent cause. If, however, the PVCs are frequent (> 6 per minute) or multiformed, they could indicate ventricular irritability, which may be caused by myocardial ischemia or infarction, congestive heart failure, hypoxia, acidosis, digitalis toxicity, or electrolyte derangements (sodium, potassium, magnesium).

Isolated PVCs in patients without underlying cardiovascular disease are usually clinically insignificant, and are typically not treated. If, however, PVCs occur in the context of a potential cardiac event, digitalis toxicity, or electrolyte disturbance, they have a greater likelihood of deteriorating to ventricular tachycardia or ventricular fibrillation and are generally treated with an antidysrhythmic agent or other therapy aimed at treating the underlying cause (eg, electrolyte replacement).

3. What is your field impression of this patient?

This patient's symptomatology indicates that he is experiencing an *addisonian crisis*. The following assessment findings support this field impression:

- **History of Addison's disease.** As its name implies, addisonian crisis is an event unique to patients with Addison's disease.
- **Temperature of 101.5° F,** which indicates an infection, a common precursor to addisonian crisis.
- **Hypoglycemia** is frequently seen in patients with addisonian crisis.
- **Altered mental status,** which indicates decreased cerebral perfusion and is likely caused by a combination of his hypoglycemia and hypotension.
- **Hypotension,** which, in patients with addisonian crisis, is caused by severe dehydration.
- **Generalized weakness,** which is likely the result of a combination of sodium and potassium depletion and hypoglycemia.
- **Premature ventricular complexes,** which could indicate an electrolyte abnormality, most notably a derangement in potassium.

In order to have an understanding of addisonian crisis, we must first set the stage by discussing the pathophysiology of Addison's disease.

Primary Addison's disease, also referred to as primary adrenocortical insufficiency, is caused by progressive destruction and/or shrinking (atrophy) of the adrenal cortex, a part of the adrenal gland. In approximately 90% of all cases, this atrophy is due to an autoimmune disorder, in which the immune system begins identifying the cells of the adrenal cortex as foreign, and produces antibodies that destroy them. Other causes of Addison's disease include tuberculosis, fungal infections, and malignancies of the adrenal cortex.

In some patients, Addison's disease is drug-induced, specifically when the patient is being treated with corticosteroids, such as prednisone, for an unrelated illness. Corticosteroids suppress normal adrenal function, and acute cessation of therapy can cause symptoms of Addison's disease and perhaps even an acute addisonian crisis.

Regardless of the underlying cause of Addison's disease, destruction of the adrenal cortex renders it unable to produce two extremely important hormones: cortisol and aldosterone.

Cortisol is a very potent hormone involved in regulating the functioning of nearly every type of organ and tissue in the body. It is considered to be one of the few hormones absolutely necessary for life, which is clear when you understand the numerous roles that it plays in the body **(Table 20-5)**.

Table 20-5 The Roles of Cortisol in the Body

The complex processing and utilization of sugar, fats, and proteins
The normal functioning of the circulatory system and the heart
The functioning of muscles
Normal kidney function
Production of blood cells
The normal processes involved in maintaining the skeletal system
Proper functioning of the brain and nerves
The normal response of the immune system

Aldosterone, also produced in the adrenal cortex, plays a central role in maintaining the appropriate proportions of salt and water in the body. When this delicate balance is upset, circulating volume throughout the body falls to dangerously low levels, causing electrolyte disturbances, profound hypotension, and cardiac dysrhythmias.

In the vast majority of cases, Addison's disease develops gradually, and the symptoms **(Table 20-6)** are not noticed until approximately 90% of the adrenal cortex has been destroyed.

Table 20-6 Symptoms of Addison's Disease

Fatigue and loss of energy
Muscle weakness
Anorexia (loss of appetite)
Weight loss
Nausea, vomiting, and diarrhea
Abdominal pain
Dehydration
Hyperpigmented skin (increased melanin production)

Addison's disease affects both men and women equally, and occurs in approximately 4 of 100,000 people. This statistic makes the disease a rare occurrence.

The prognosis for patients with Addison's disease is surprisingly good, provided they are appropriately treated. If however, the disease is not treated, or the treatment is substandard, the patient is at high risk for complications, most notably addisonian crisis.

Addisonian crisis is an acute exacerbation of Addison's disease often precipitated by an acute stressor such as a severe illness, infection, or trauma. Because the acute stressor overwhelms the adrenal cortex and significantly reduces the production of cortisol and aldosterone, Addisonian crisis can, and often does, occur in patients who are being appropriately and otherwise effectively treated for Addison's disease.

Addisonian crisis causes a variety of problems for the patient. Blood glucose levels fall dangerously low (hypoglycemia), which produces its own set of problems. In addition, the kidneys excrete excessive amounts of sodium (hyponatremia), resulting in severe dehydration and profound hypotension. Potassium retention (hyperkalemia) also occurs, which predisposes the patient to potentially life-threatening cardiac dysrhythmias, such as ventricular tachycardia or ventricular fibrillation. Hyperkalemia-induced ventricular dysrhythmias are often the result of an R-on-T phenomenon, in which an ectopic ventricular pacemaker depolarizes before the prior cardiac cycle's repolarization phase is complete.

You should maintain a high index of suspicion for addisonian crisis in patients with sudden, unexplained cardiovascular collapse, especially if there is a history of primary Addison's disease, or Addison's secondary to drug therapy (prednisone).

4. Are the patient's vital signs and SAMPLE history consistent with your field impression?

This patient's hypotension indicates severe dehydration, which is experienced in addisonian crisis. His heart rate, however, which would be expected to be rapid, is normal because of a lack of adrenal hormones. In fact, many patients with addisonian crisis are initially seen with bradycardia. The patient's rapid, shallow breathing is a sign of shock secondary to the acute crisis.

In addition to the history of Addison's disease, the preceding events are a classic precursor to addisonian crisis. The recent infection is the most likely cause of his crisis. Severe illness or infection is perhaps one of the most common causes of addisonian crisis. The patient's medications are ones commonly prescribed to patients with Addison's disease.

■ **Hydrocortisone** (Cortef) is a naturally occurring corticosteroid (glucocortocoid-type) used in the treatment of Addison's disease.

■ **Fludrocortisone acetate** (Florinef) is a mineralcorticoid that produces marked sodium retention and inhibits excess adrenocortical secretion. Florinef is also used in the treatment of Addison's disease.

5. What specific treatment is required for this patient's condition?

■ **50% dextrose**
  • Although you have already given the patient one 25-g dose of dextrose, you should administer another 25 g because his blood glucose level remains less than 60 mg/dL and he is still symptomatic (eg, disoriented). Hypoglycemia poses its own threat to life, and must be treated immediately.

■ **Aggressive fluid resuscitation**
  • This patient's hypotension is caused by profound dehydration and must be treated with IV fluid boluses. Administration of 20 mL/kg of normal saline is a typical dose for hypovolemic patients. However, this patient will likely require more aggressive fluid boluses.

If IV fluids do not raise the patient's blood pressure enough to improve tissue perfusion, vasopressor drugs (eg, dopamine, epinephrine) may be needed. Follow locally established protocols or contact medical control as needed regarding vasopressor therapy.

Prompt transport is essential, as definitive treatment for this patient will require correcting sodium deficiency, rehydration, and the administration of corticosteroids.

6. Is further treatment required for this patient?

With aggressive fluid resuscitation, you have improved the patient's blood pressure and further administration of 50% dextrose has markedly improved his mental status. The combination of increased tissue perfusion and correction of his hypoglycemia has also resulted in improved respirations.

Further management at this point should consist of continuous monitoring of airway, breathing, and circulation. Continue to observe his cardiac rhythm, as he is still at risk for cardiac dysrhythmias.

7. Are there any special considerations for this patient?

Although you have stabilized this patient's condition and prevented imminent cardiovascular collapse, he is still in need of definitive care, which will consist of administering corticosteroids and correction of electrolyte abnormalities. Until these therapies can be provided, the patient is still at risk for a rebound to his original condition. It is therefore of extreme importance that you continuously monitor his condition for signs of deterioration and be prepared to treat him accordingly.

Summary

Addison's disease is a rare condition characterized by destruction of the adrenal cortex and subsequent failure in the production of cortisol and aldosterone, both of which are hormones vital in the normal functioning of numerous body systems.

Primary Addison's disease is caused by progressive destruction of the adrenal cortex and is most commonly the result of an autoimmune disorder. Addison's disease can also be drug-induced, when the patient is taking prednisone, a steroid that suppresses adrenal function. Abrupt cessation of prednisone therapy can trigger symptoms of Addison's disease.

Addisonian crisis is an acute exacerbation of Addison's disease that is commonly preceded by an infection, severe illness, trauma, or any other stressor that requires increased adrenal function.

The symptoms of addisonian crisis are related to the depletion of blood glucose and sodium, and the retention of potassium. As a result, the patient often experiences hypoglycemia, severe dehydration and hypotension, and cardiac dysrhythmias.

Management for a patient with addisonian crisis begins by establishing a patent airway and ensuring adequate oxygenation and ventilation. Positive pressure ventilatory support may be required if the patient is breathing inadequately.

Further treatment consists of administering 25 to 50 g of 50% dextrose if the patient's blood glucose level is less than 60 mg/dL and aggressive fluid resuscitation to improve blood pressure and tissue perfusion. Prompt transport to definitive care is essential.